QUICK GUIDE TO ENDOCRINOLOGY

QUICK GUIDE TO ENDOCRINOLOGY

The Pediatric Version

SECOND EDITION

LAURA M JACOBSEN

Assistant Professor, Departments of Pediatrics and Pathology,
Immunology and Laboratory Medicine, University of Florida
Diabetes Institute, University of Florida, Gainesville, FL,
United States
Associate Program Director, Pediatric Endocrinology
Fellowship, University of Florida, Gainesville, FL, United States

BRITTANY S BRUGGEMAN

Assistant Professor, Department of Pediatrics, University
of Florida Diabetes Institute, University of Florida, Gainesville,
FL, United States

WILLIAM E WINTER

Professor, Departments of Pathology, Immunology and
Laboratory Medicine, Pediatrics, and Molecular Genetics and
Microbiology, University of Florida Diabetes Institute,
University of Florida, Gainesville, FL, United States

First Edition published by ADLM previously known as AACC

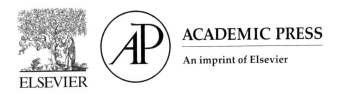

ELSEVIER

ACADEMIC PRESS
An imprint of Elsevier

Academic Press is an imprint of Elsevier
125 London Wall, London EC2Y 5AS, United Kingdom
525 B Street, Suite 1650, San Diego, CA 92101, United States
50 Hampshire Street, 5th Floor, Cambridge, MA 02139, United States

Notices

Knowledge and best practice in this field are constantly changing. As new research and experience broaden our understanding, changes in research methods, professional practices, or medical treatment may become necessary.

Practitioners and researchers must always rely on their own experience and knowledge in evaluating and using any information, methods, compounds, or experiments described herein. In using such information or methods they should be mindful of their own safety and the safety of others, including parties for whom they have a professional responsibility.

To the fullest extent of the law, neither the Publisher nor the authors, contributors, or editors, assume any liability for any injury and/or damage to persons or property as a matter of products liability, negligence or otherwise, or from any use or operation of any methods, products, instructions, or ideas contained in the material herein.

ISBN 978-0-443-14135-5

For information on all Academic Press publications
visit our website at https://www.elsevier.com/books-and-journals

Publisher: Stacy Masucci
Acquisitions Editor: Patricia M. Osborn
Editorial Project Manager: Sara Pianavilla
Production Project Manager: Jayadivya Saiprasad
Cover Designer: Mark Rogers

Typeset by STRAIVE, India

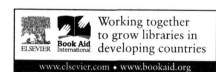

Working together
to grow libraries in
developing countries

www.elsevier.com • www.bookaid.org

Contents

Abbreviations

Hormones

1,25-OH2D	1,25-dihydroxyvitamin D
25-OHD	25-hydroxyvitamin D
ACTH	adrenocorticotropic hormone
ADH	antidiuretic hormone
ALS	acid-labile subunit
AMH	Müllerian-inhibiting hormone (anti-Müllerian hormone)
CNS	central nervous system
CRH	corticotropin-releasing hormone
DHEA-S	dehydroepiandrosterone sulfate
DHT	dihydrotestosterone
FSH	follicle-stimulating hormone
GH	growth hormone
GHRH	growth hormone-releasing hormone
GnRH	gonadotropin-releasing hormone
HCG	human chorionic gonadotropin
IGF-1	insulin-like growth factor 1 (somatomedin C)
IGF-BP3	insulin-like growth factor binding protein 3
LH	luteinizing hormone
PRIH	prolactin-release-inhibiting hormone
Prl	prolactin
PTH	parathyroid hormone
PTHrP	parathyroid hormone-related peptide
SRIH	somatotropin release-inhibiting hormone (somatostatin)
TRH	thyrotropin-releasing hormone
TSH	thyrotropin-stimulating hormone

Other

AITD	autoimmune thyroid disease
APS	autoimmune polyglandular syndrome
AT	atrophic thyroiditis
BP	binding protein
CAH	congenital adrenal hyperplasia
DCT	distal convoluted tubule
DDAVP	1-desamino-8-D-arginine vasopressin (desmopressin)
DI	diabetes insipidus
DM	diabetes mellitus
DSD	difference of sexual development
GD	Graves disease

GHD	growth hormone deficiency
GV	growth velocity
HT	Hashimoto thyroiditis
PRA	plasma renin activity
SIADH	syndrome of inappropriate antidiuretic hormone
TBII	thyrotropin-binding inhibitory immunoglobulin
Tg	thyroglobulin
TPO	thyroperoxidase
TSI	thyroid-stimulating immunoglobulin

CHAPTER 1

Introduction to pediatric endocrinology

Scope of text

As an update to the "Quick Guide to Endocrinology" (American Association for Clinical Chemistry Press, 2013), this text focuses on practical pediatric endocrinology. We will explore not only physiology, but also diagnostic and measurement challenges for endocrinological disorders. The intended audience is trainees and practitioners in the fields of pediatric endocrinology, general pediatrics, family medicine, pathology, and clinical chemistry including fellows, residents, medical students, nursing students, and advance practice provider students. The reader will learn from this book, in an easy to read, quick format, the physiology and method of measurement for hormones essential to bodily processes and how their dysregulation results in disease. The characteristics of such diseases and diagnostic testing including up-to-date molecular assays and emerging measurement interferences are a valuable resource for those in the medical field.

Definition and description of hormones

- Hormones are chemical messengers used by the endocrine system.
  - The secreted messenger (Fig. 1.1):
    - Enters the interstitium;
    - Diffuses into the circulation; and
    - Exits the circulation into the interstitium at a distant site to bind to a cell receptor (either located on the cellular plasma membrane or located in the cell cytoplasm).

Quick Guide to Endocrinology
https://doi.org/10.1016/B978-0-443-14135-5.00007-7

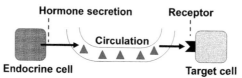

Fig. 1.1 In endocrine systems, the endocrine cell secretes its hormone product (triangles) into the interstitial fluid, which immediately bathes the cell. Through diffusion down a simple concentration gradient, the hormone enters the bloodstream to systemically circulate. Plasma-binding proteins for the hormone may or may not exist. At the distal tissues, again by diffusion down a simple concentration gradient, the hormone enters the interstitium. Cells that express a receptor for the hormone can then respond to the hormone. Although this illustration is drawn with the receptor on the surface, the receptor could be intracellular or could be expressed both intracellularly and on the plasma membrane.

- In the endocrine system, chemical messengers are typically (1) steroid hormones derived from cholesterol or (2) composed of amino acids which can be grouped by size (single amino acids, peptides, polypeptides, and proteins) and receptor type (G-protein coupled receptor [GPCR], nuclear receptor, tyrosine kinase receptor, and type 1 cytokine receptor) (Table 1.1). In the case of steroid hormones, they are comprised of a modified gonane structure (four hydrocarbon rings fused together) derived from cholesterol and are small molecules.

Table 1.1 Endocrine hormones organized by their structural components, relative size, and receptor type.

Class	Example	No. AA/Relative Size	Receptor Type
Proteins	GH, prolactin	191-199	Type 1 cytokine
Glycoproteins	LH(CG), FSH, TSH	α 92 β 111-145	GPCR
Polypeptides	PTH	84	GPCR
	Insulin, IGF-1	51-70	Tyrosine kinase
	CRH, GnRH, GHRH	38-56	GPCR
	ACTH	39	GPCR
	Glucagon, somatostatin	14-30	GPCR
Peptides (oligopeptide)	ADH (binds V2 receptor)	9	GPCR
	TRH	3	GPCR
Single AA Derivatives	Dopamine	1	GPCR
	Catecholamines	1	GPCR
	Thyroid hormone	1	Nuclear receptor
Steroid Hormones	Mineralocorticoids		Nuclear receptor
	Glucocorticoids	Cholesterol derivative	Nuclear receptor
	Sex Steroids		Nuclear receptor
Sterols	Vitamin D3		Nuclear receptor

GPCR, G-protein coupled receptor

- Many systems of the body use chemical messengers (Table 1.2).

Table 1.2 Systems of the body that use chemical messengers.

System	Examples	System type
Nervous	Neurotransmitter	Paracrine
Immune	Cytokines	Paracrine
		Autocrine
		Endocrine (least common)
Gastrointestinal tract	Gastrin	Endocrine
Erythropoietic	Erythropoietin	Endocrine
Thrombopoietic	Thrombopoietin	Endocrine
Maintenance of iron balance	Hepcidin	Endocrine
Hepcidin regulation	IL-6; erythroferrone	Endocrine

- Steroid hormones, for example, are made and secreted from the adrenal cortex, gonads, and placenta and act on other target organs; their precursor is cholesterol (Fig. 1.2).
  - One such steroid hormone, DHEA-S, is the most abundant circulating hormone in the body.

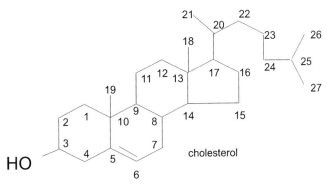

Fig. 1.2 Cholesterol is the building block for steroid hormones, including mineralocorticoids, glucocorticoids, adrenal androgens, testosterone, estrogens, and progesterone.

- Some hormones also function as neurotransmitters and some are produced at more than one site in the body (e.g., somatostatin).

- ○ The hypothalamus secretes somatostatin to suppress the release of growth hormone (GH) from the anterior pituitary gland (Fig. 1.3).
- ○ Delta cells of the islets of Langerhans secrete somatostatin to suppress both glucagon and insulin secretion (Fig. 1.4).

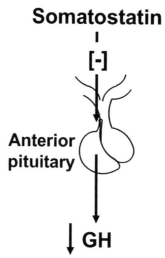

Fig. 1.3 Somatostatin secreted by the hypothalamus suppresses the release of growth hormone (GH) from the anterior pituitary gland.

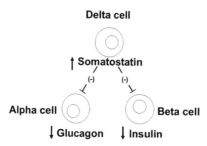

Fig. 1.4 Somatostatin secreted by the delta cells of the islets of Langerhans suppresses the release of insulin from beta cells and the release of glucagon from alpha cells.

- • In paracrine systems, the secreted messenger binds to a cell receptor on an adjacent cell (Fig. 1.5).
  - ○ E.g., the secretion of insulin by beta cells suppresses the secretion of glucagon from alpha cells that are also located within the islets of Langerhans (Fig. 1.6).

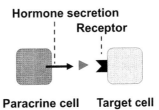

Fig. 1.5 In paracrine systems, the endocrine cell and the target cell are only separated by interstitial fluid and are immediately adjacent to one another. Similar to Fig. 1.2, although this figure is drawn with the receptor on the surface, the receptor could be intracellular or could be expressed both intracellularly and on the plasma membrane.

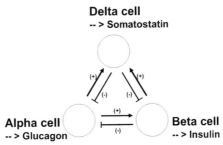

Fig. 1.6 The islets of Langerhans in the pancreas use paracrine systems to balance insulin and glucagon secretion to maintain glucose homeostasis, thus resisting the development of both hypoglycemia and hyperglycemia. Glucagon stimulates the release of insulin, whereas insulin suppresses glucagon. Somatostatin is stimulated by both insulin and glucagon and, in turn, suppresses both insulin and glucagon.

- In the nervous system, the anatomy of a paracrine interaction is described as a synapse (Fig. 1.7).

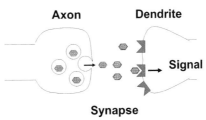

Fig. 1.7 The synapse is the anatomic and neurochemical junction between "upstream" axons that convey electrical signals via neurotransmitters to "downstream" dendrites that express receptors for the neurotransmitters.

- In autocrine systems, the secreted messenger binds to a receptor on the cell that secreted that messenger (Fig. 1.8).
  - E.g., the secretion of interleukin (IL)-2 by an activated CD4 T cell binds to IL-2 receptors on that same cell, thus stimulating the cell to proliferate (Fig. 1.9).

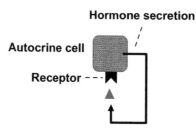

Fig. 1.8 In autocrine systems, the endocrine cell responds to its own hormonal product (triangle) secreted into the interstitium.

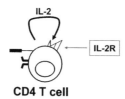

Fig. 1.9 An example of an autocrine system where a CD4 T cell produces and responds to interleukin-2 (IL-2) via the expression of the IL-2 receptor.

Hormone secretion and transport

- In endocrine glands, the hormone:
  - Is released into the interstitial fluid, which surrounds the endocrine cell; and
  - Diffuses into the circulation for systemic distribution (Fig. 1.10).

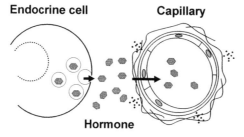

Fig. 1.10 Hormones secreted by endocrine cells diffuse into the interstitium to then enter into the circulation.

- In turn, the cells (in the target organs) that express hormone receptors respond to the hormone.
- By contrast, in exocrine glands, the secretory product:
  - Enters a duct to exit the exocrine gland to enter a cavity (e.g., gastrointestinal tract); or
  - Is released onto the skin (e.g., through sweat, breast milk) (Fig. 1.11).

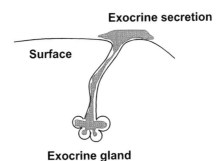

Fig. 1.11 Exocrine cells secrete their products into the lumens of tubes that are connected to a surface. Illustrated is a simple cartoon of a sweat gland.

- Some hormones are "carried" in the circulation and are bound to binding proteins.
  - In such cases, the free, unbound hormone appears to be the biologically active form of the hormone (Fig. 1.12).

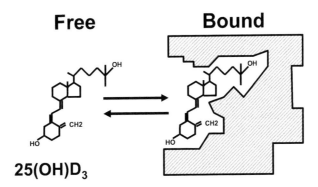

Fig. 1.12 Some hormones circulate in both free and bound states when there is a transport protein for the hormone. Illustrated is 25-hydroxyvitamin D_3 and vitamin D binding protein.

- Hormones and their binding proteins are listed in Table 1.3. Various disease states may alter the concentration of binding proteins (e.g., nephrotic syndrome) and must be considered when choosing an assay.

Table 1.3 Hormones and their binding proteins.

Hormone	Binding proteins
T4, T3	Thyroxine-binding globulin (TBG), thyroxine-binding prealbumin (TBPA; transthyretin), albumin
Testosterone, estradiol	Sex hormone-binding globulin (SHBG); albumin
Cortisol	Cortisol-binding globulin (transcortin)
GH	GH-binding protein
IGF-1	IGF-BP3 plus the acid-labile subunit (ALS)
Calcitriol	Vitamin D binding protein (VDBP)
ADH	Neurophysins

T4, thyroxine; T3, tri-iodothyronine; GH, growth hormone; IGF-1, insulin-like growth factor-1; ADH, anti-diuretic hormone.

- Some carrier proteins are derived from the extracellular domain of the hormone's cell surface receptor.
    - E.g., GH-binding protein (Fig. 1.13).

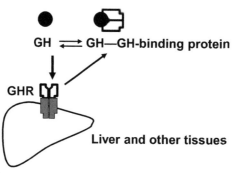

Fig. 1.13 The binding protein for a hormone can be a part of its receptor. Illustrated here is growth hormone (GH) and its binding protein (GH-binding protein) that is part of the GH receptor (GHR).

- Examples of hormones where free hormone measurements are used clinically include:
    - Free thyroxine (T4);
    - Free 3,5,3'-tri-iodothyronine (T3); and
    - Free testosterone.

Hormone actions

- Hormones can have multiple actions, e.g.:
  - Insulin stimulates glycolysis, glycogen synthesis, fatty acid synthesis, triglyceride synthesis, and protein synthesis; and
  - Insulin also suppresses glycogenolysis, gluconeogenesis, and ketogenesis.
- Multiple hormones can have similar actions.
  - E.g., epinephrine, glucagon, cortisol, and GH all raise the level of plasma glucose (Fig. 1.14).

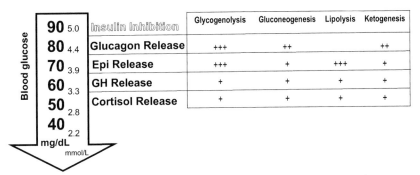

Blood glucose			Glycogenolysis	Gluconeogenesis	Lipolysis	Ketogenesis
90 5.0	Insulin Inhibition					
80 4.4	Glucagon Release		+++	++		++
70 3.9	Epi Release		+++	+	+++	+
60 3.3	GH Release		+	+	+	+
50 2.8	Cortisol Release		+	+	+	+
40 2.2	mg/dL mmol/L					

Fig. 1.14 Multiple hormones can have the same action. Illustrated here is the concept that epinephrine, glucagon, cortisol, and growth hormone all raise plasma glucose concentrations. The release of these counter-regulatory hormones is stimulated at different levels of hypoglycemia and act through various mechanisms to increase plasma glucose.

- Hormones act by binding to cell receptors.
  - Cell receptors for protein hormones and catecholamines exist on cell surfaces (Fig. 1.15).

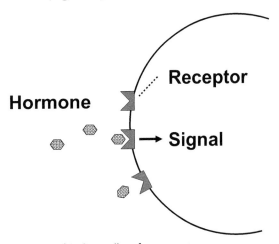

Fig. 1.15 Some hormones bind to cell-surface receptors.

- o Cell receptors for steroid hormones and thyroid hormones are intra-cellular (Fig. 1.16).

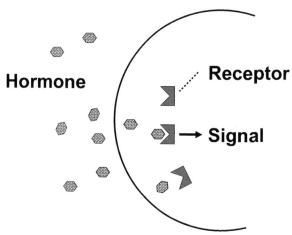

Fig. 1.16 Some hormones bind to cytoplasmic receptors.

- Intracellular steroid hormone receptors may also be expressed on the cell surface.
  - o This explains the rapid actions of some hormones previously known to bind to intracellular receptors (e.g., thyroid hormone, cortisol).
- In general, responses to protein hormones and catecholamines are rapid
  - o E.g., minutes to hours to days
- Responses to steroid hormones and thyroid hormones may be acute and chronic
  - o E.g., days to weeks to months
- Hormones that bind to cell-surface receptors trigger the generation of second messengers.
  - o E.g., cyclic adenosine monophosphate (cAMP), phospholipase C
- When hormones bind to receptors (G-protein coupled receptors) that ultimately lead to the generation of cAMP, the hormone-receptor complex interacts with a G protein (Fig. 1.17).

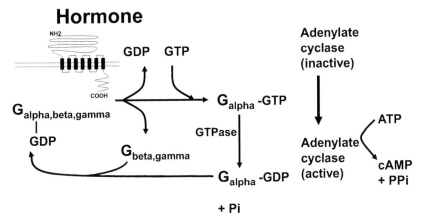

Hormone

Fig. 1.17 One important example of a second messenger system involves the generation of cAMP. After a hormone binds to its receptor, the receptor changes conformation and can interact with the G stimulatory protein that is composed of three subunits: alpha, beta, and gamma. The alpha subunit separates from the beta and gamma subunits. GDP on the G alpha subunit is replaced by GTP, thus allowing the G alpha subunit to activate AC. AC converts ATP to cAMP plus PPi. G alpha-GTP acquires GTPase activity cleaving a Pi from GTP, thus producing GDP. G alpha-GDP cannot activate AC. Subsequently, G stimulatory protein in its basal form is reconstituted as G alpha-GDP and binds to G beta and G gamma. Interestingly, in McCune-Albright syndrome, a loss-of-function mutation in the G alpha that impairs its normal GTPase activity (when G alpha-GTP is present) leads to persistent activation of AC, producing, for example, precocious puberty, hyperthyroidism, polyostotic fibrous dysplasia, and more. cAMP, cyclic adenosine monophosphate; GDP, guanosine diphosphate; GTP, guanosine triphosphate; AC, adenyl cyclase; ATP, adenosine triphosphate; PPi, pyrophosphate; Pi, phosphate.

Hormone regulation

- Negative feedback networks control most hormones.
- The negative feedback signal may be supplied by:
  - Another hormone (Fig. 1.18), the original hormone itself (i.e. in the case of prolactin's inhibition of its own release); or
  - Alteration in the concentration of a regulated metabolic molecule such as glucose or an ion such as ionized calcium (Fig. 1.19).

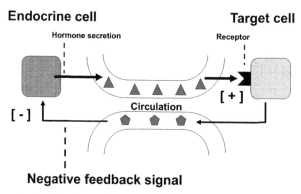

Fig. 1.18 Negative feedback in endocrine systems can be achieved when the target cell produces a hormone (pentagons) that is detected by the endocrine cell, thus reducing the secretion of the regulatory hormone (triangles). For example, the anterior pituitary corticotrophs secrete ACTH which stimulates the adrenal cortex to secrete cortisol. Cortisol, in a negative feedback loop, inhibits the anterior pituitary secretion of ACTH.

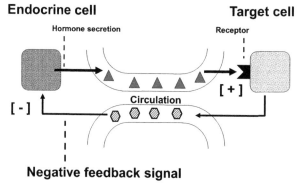

Fig. 1.19 Negative feedback in endocrine systems can also be achieved when the target cell (e.g., hepatocyte) produces a metabolic molecule (e.g., glucose [hexagons]) that is detected by the endocrine cell, thus reducing the secretion of the regulatory hormone (triangles). For example, if glucose levels decline, then glucagon is secreted. Glucagon then acts on the liver to increase glucose production through glycogenolysis and gluconeogenesis.

- Rarely, positive feedback controls hormone secretion.
    - During the luteinizing hormone (LH) surge in the midcycle of the menstrual cycle, which stimulates ovulation, the LH rises because of the increase in estradiol levels that are being increased by LH (Fig. 1.20).

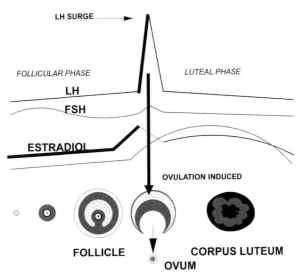

Fig. 1.20 Positive feedback loops do exist. For example, in the late follicular phase, estrogen stimulates luteinizing hormone (LH) secretion leading to an LH surge and subsequent ovulation.

- Hormones are classified differently depending on whether they are controlled or not controlled by the hypothalamus and pituitary gland.
- Several hormones are controlled by the hypothalamus and anterior pituitary gland (Fig. 1.21).
- Hormones synthesized in the hypothalamus and secreted by the posterior pituitary gland (Fig. 1.22) include:
    ○ Arginine vasopressin, also known as vasopressin or anti-diuretic hormone (ADH); and
    ○ Oxytocin.
- While several hormones are controlled by the hypothalamic–pituitary axis, several hormones are not controlled by this axis (Table 1.4).

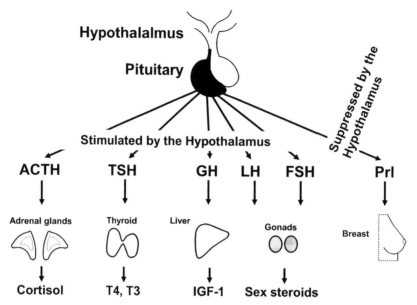

Fig. 1.21 Most hormones secreted by the anterior pituitary gland are regulated solely or predominantly by stimulation (i.e., ACTH, TSH, GH, LH, FSH), whereas only Prl is regulated by suppression (i.e., by dopamine that acts as a Prl release-inhibiting hormone). These pituitary hormones stimulate their target organs for the release of another messenger in most cases (i.e., Cortisol, T4, T3, IGF-1, Sex Steroids). ACTH, adrenocorticotropic hormone; TSH, thyroid-stimulating hormone; GH, growth hormone; LH, luteinizing hormone; FSH, follicle-stimulating hormone; Prl, prolactin; T4, thyroxine; T3, 3,5,3′-tri-iodothyronine; IGF-1, insulin-like growth factor-1.

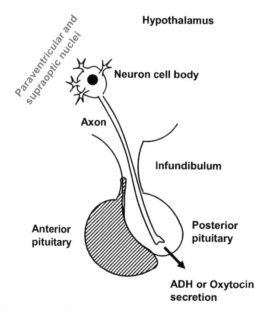

Fig. 1.22 Posterior pituitary gland hormones are synthesized in the neuronal cell bodies in the hypothalamus. Axons from these neurons extend though the pituitary stalk into the posterior pituitary gland where hormone secretion occurs. ADH, anti-diuretic hormone.

Table 1.4 Hormones not controlled by the hypothalamus and pituitary gland.

Insulin
Glucagon
Epinephrine
Aldosterone
Parathyroid hormone
Calcitonin
Gastrointestinal tract hormones (e.g., gastrin, secretin, cholecystokinin, incretin)
Thymosin (thymic hormones involved in T-cell development)

Manifestations of endocrine disorders

- There are four general types of perturbations that can affect the endocrine system:
  1. Hypofunction;
  2. Hyperfunction;
  3. Disturbed hormone secretion related to nonendocrine disease (physiologic and pathologic); and
  4. Endocrine tumors.
- Although most tumors do not involve the over- or undersecretion of hormone, some tumors are endocrinologically active and may produce symptoms.
  - E.g., pheochromocytoma (producing catecholamine excess), toxic thyroid adenoma (causing hyperthyroidism)
- Disturbed hormone secretion related to nonendocrine disease can be physiologic.
  - E.g., when transient hypercortisolism and catecholamine excess occurs in response to stress (Fig. 1.23)

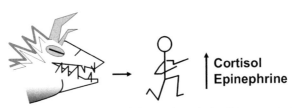

Cortisol
Epinephrine

Fig. 1.23 In response to stress, epinephrine and cortisol will be secreted.

- Disturbed hormone secretion related to nonendocrine disease can be pathologic.
    - ○ Hypogonadism and infertility can occur in response to (1) stress, (2) weight loss, (3) states of insulin resistance, or (4) as a result of alkylating chemotherapeutic agents.
- Sick euthyroid syndrome (e.g., nonthyroidal illness) can lower the T3 level in states of severe acute or chronic illness (Fig. 1.24). This is an appropriate, compensatory mechanism. Most experts believe that sick euthyroid syndrome should not be treated with thyroxine.

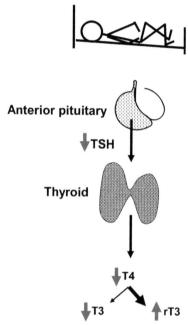

Fig. 1.24 With prolonged sick euthyroid syndrome due to severe illness in hospitalized patients, TSH can decline, leading to a fall in T4 concentration and consequently a fall in T3 by shunting to rT3.

- Endocrine tumors may or may not be neoplasms.
    - ○ "Masses" (i.e., tumors) in endocrine glands that are not neoplasms include hyperplasias and cysts.
- Endocrine neoplasms may be benign or malignant.
    - ○ Malignancy is indicated when (Fig. 1.25):
        - ▪ A neoplasm spreads outside of the gland of origin (e.g., a capsule is breached by the tumor);

- Blood vessels are invaded; or
- There are metastases in lymph nodes or metastases to distant tissues or organs.
  - In some endocrine neoplasms, the histology can clearly indicate malignancy.
    - E.g., nuclear appearance of a papillary thyroid carcinoma is pathognomonic
  - In other neoplasms, the histology—even if bizarre in appearance—may not indicate malignancy.
    - E.g., pheochromocytoma

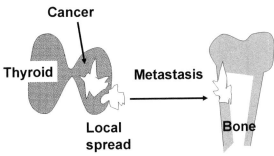

Fig. 1.25 As illustrated in the case of thyroid cancer, evidence of malignancy includes local invasion, invasion of blood vessels, and/or distant metastasis.

Hormone and molecular assays

- Hormone levels are measured in large part using immunoassays (biochemical tests to detect and measure proteins, steroids, amino acid derivatives or other substances using antibodies) which include:
  - Competitive assays, for small hormones (e.g., free T4). These measure the amount of the labeled "competitor" left bound to antibody after the hormone from the patient's sera displaces it (Fig. 1.26).
    - Measured competitor is inversely related, in a hyperbolic fashion, to hormone quantity (Fig. 1.27).
  - Non-competitive assays, for large hormones (e.g., TSH). These measure the amount of signal (e.g., fluorescence) when both the capture and detection antibodies have bound to the hormone from the patient's sera (Fig. 1.28).

○ Hormone is measure directly ("sandwiched" between two antibodies) and is linearly related to hormone quantity (Fig. 1.27).

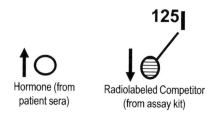

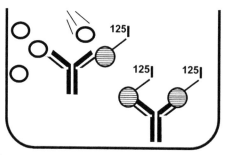

Fig. 1.26 For small hormones, a competitive assay uses a fixed amount of antibody (that binds the hormone of interest) and a competitor (analyte) that also binds the antibody. As the hormone level goes up, more of its binds to the antibody, displacing the competitor, and the level of bound competitor goes down.

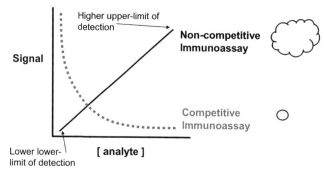

Fig. 1.27 Sandwich, non-competitive, assays produce a signal (e.g., luminescence) proportional to the amount of hormone. Measurement occurs when labeled antibody binds to hormone. Conversely, for competitive immunoassays, measurement occurs when the patient's hormone displaces the labeled hormone (competitor). This results in an inverse relationship; as the patient's hormone level increases, less of the labeled hormone (competitor) is able to bind to the detection antibody.

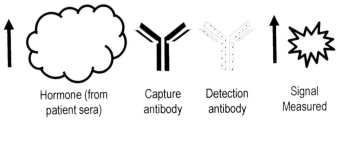

Hormone (from patient sera)   Capture antibody   Detection antibody   Signal Measured

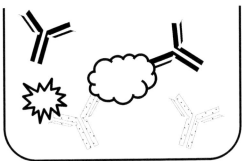

Fig. 1.28 For large hormones, non-competitive assays are ideal. A capture and a detection antibody sandwich the large hormone releasing a signal that is measured. The more hormone present, the more signal detected.

- As with any laboratory test, interactions or interferences may occur that limit the accuracy of the measurement that include (Table 1.5):
    - Pre-analytical;
    - Analytical;
    - Post-analytical.
- Assays may have patient preparation steps including posture and avoidance of contraindicated medications (e.g., plasma renin activity and plasma metanephrines, respectively).
- Finally, in this text we will also introduce molecular testing which is the sequencing of DNA or RNA to predict disease:
    - Some examples in pediatric endocrinology include genetics variants in: *CYP21A2* (classical congenital adrenal hyperplasia—21-hydroxylase deficiency); *VDR* (vitamin D resistance rickets); *RET* proto-oncogene (multiple endocrine neoplasia [MEN] 2); *SDHB* (familial paraganglioma syndrome).
    - If high suspicion for a genetic syndrome or hereditary disease, specific genes or gene panels may shed light on the diagnosis.

Table 1.5 Hormone assay interferences can occur before, during, and after the analytical processing of a patient's sample.

Class of interference	Example
Pre-analytical	Wrong patient
	Wrong patient positioning (e.g., sitting versus recumbent)
	Wrong time of day
	Wrong tube
	Wrong volume of blood
	Inappropriate storage (e.g., wrong temperature) and processing
Analytical	Lack of assay specificity (e.g., cortisol assay detects many different glucocorticoids)
	Poor low-end sensitivity (e.g., testosterone immunoassay unable to detect under 200 ng/dL)
	High-dose hook effect in the prolactin immunoassay (see Chapter 2)
	Macro-complexes (e.g., prolactin—anti-prolactin antibody complexes) (see Chapter 2)
	False positive due to human anti-mouse, rheumatoid factor, or heterophile antibodies
	Biotin[a] interference
Post-analytical	Wrong result reported in patient's chart
	Results misinterpreted by ordering physician, e.g., using a reference range of different units, not considering the status of binding proteins in the blood, or failure to consider analyte half-life or pulsatile release

[a]A B vitamin (B7) is used in complex with streptavidin coated to a magnetic particle for quantification. Biotin ingested at high doses (found in hair/nail supplements) can falsely elevate competitive immunoassays (e.g., free T4 elevation) and falsely lower non-competitive immunoassays (e.g., lower TSH).

Suggested reading

Jacobsen LM, Bazydlo LAL, Harris NS, Winter WE. Challenges in endocrinology testing. In: Dasgupta A, Sepulveda JL, editors. Accurate results in the clinical laboratory. 2nd ed. Elsevier; 2019. p. 165–89, ISBN:9780128137765. https://doi.org/10.1016/B978-0-12-813776-5.00011-X [chapter 11].

Sprague JE, Arbeláez AM. Glucose counterregulatory responses to hypoglycemia. Pediatr Endocrinol Rev 2011;9(1):463–73. quiz 474–475 PMID: 22783644. PMCID: PMC3755377.

Styne DM. Pediatric endocrinology—a clinical handbook. Cham: Springer; 2023. https://doi.org/10.1007/978-3-031-09512-2.

Winter WE, Sokoll LJ, Jialal I, editors. Handbook of diagnostic endocrinology. 3rd ed. Washington, DC: AACC Press; 2013.

CHAPTER 2

Pituitary gland

- The pituitary gland is composed of the (Figs. 2.1 and 2.2):
  o Adenohypophysis (the anterior pituitary); and
  o Neurohypophysis (the posterior pituitary).
- The anterior and posterior pituitaries are embryologically and functionally distinct.
- During fetal development, the anterior pituitary migrates to its typical location anterior to the posterior pituitary.
  o Adenohypophysis is derived from oral ectoderm
- The posterior pituitary gland is an extension of the brain (Figs. 2.1 and 2.2).
  o Neurohypophysis is derived from neuroectoderm

Anterior pituitary
Physiology
- Products of the anterior pituitary gland and their relative location and size within the gland include (Fig. 2.3):
  o Thyrotrophs (15% of total cell mass of anterior pituitary) secrete thyroid-stimulating hormone (TSH; discussed further in Chapter 3);
  o Corticotrophs (15%) secrete adrenal corticotrophic hormone (ACTH, also known as corticotropin; discussed further Chapter 4);
  o Somatotrophs (45%) secrete growth hormone (GH);
  o Gonadotrophs (10%) secrete both luteinizing hormone (LH) and follicle-stimulating hormone (FSH; both discussed further in Chapter 5); and
  o Lactotrophs (15%) secrete prolactin (Prl).
- The anterior pituitary hormones are either controlled by (Fig. 2.4):
  o Hypothalamic stimulatory-releasing hormones (TSH, ACTH, LH, and FSH);
  o Release-inhibiting hormones (prolactin); or
  o A combination of both (GH).

Quick Guide to Endocrinology
https://doi.org/10.1016/B978-0-443-14135-5.00003-X

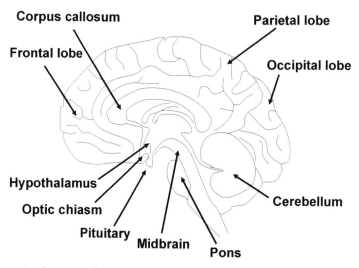

Fig. 2.1 Lateral section of the brain displaying lobes of the cerebrum (frontal, parietal, and occipital), the cerebellum, and brain stem (midbrain and pons) in reference to the hypothalamus, pituitary gland, and optic chiasm.

Prolactin

- Prolactin is secreted by anterior pituitary lactotrophs (also known as mammotrophs; Fig. 2.5) and can suppress its own release.
- Secretion is under suppressive control by dopamine released by the hypothalamus. In this setting, dopamine is known as a prolactin-release inhibiting hormone (PRIH).
- Dopamine reaches the anterior pituitary via the hypothalamic-pituitary portal system (Fig. 2.6).
- Dopamine deficiency or interruption in its delivery to the anterior pituitary because of disease of the hypothalamic-pituitary portal system will allow prolactin levels to rise.
- The action of prolactin is to support lactation from the post-partum breast.
  - Levels rise during pregnancy to help prepare the breast for lactation.
- In the postpartum period, prolactin suppresses the resumption of ovulation.
  - Continued breastfeeding does not permanently delay the resumption of menses and fertility.
  - If pregnancy is not desired during this time, then contraceptive measures should be recommended for women who are sexually active.
- During times of stress, prolactin will physiologically increase.

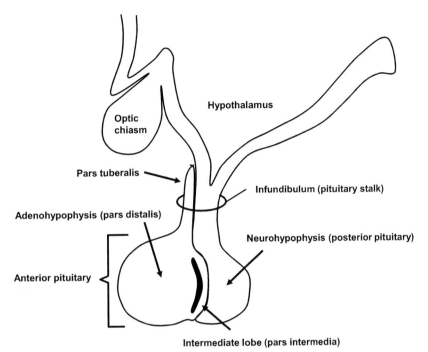

Fig. 2.2 Detailed schematic view of the hypothalamus, anterior and posterior pituitaries, and optic chiasm. The anterior pituitary is constituted by the adenohypophysis (pars distalis), the intermediate lobe (pars intermedia), and the pars tuberalis, which partially wraps around the junction of the inferior hypothalamus and the neurohypophysis (posterior pituitary). This junction and the pars tuberalis constitute the infundibulum (pituitary stalk). The adenohypophysis is active in hormone secretion. The neurohypophyseal hormones are synthesized in the hypothalamus. The pars intermedia is responsible for producing melanocyte stimulating hormone (MSH) in the fetus but is small to absent in adults.

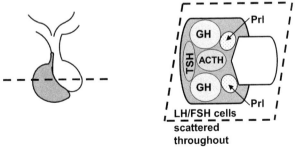

Fig. 2.3 Location and size of the cells in the anterior pituitary are pre-determined and a transverse view is indicated by the dashed line.

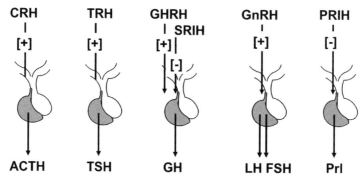

CRH	TRH	GHRH	GnRH	PRIH
[+]	[+]	[+] SRIH [-]	[+]	[-]
ACTH	TSH	GH	LH FSH	Prl

Fig. 2.4 The regulation of the anterior pituitary hormones is depicted. CRH stimulates ACTH release. TRH stimulates TSH release. GHRH stimulates GH release whereas SRIH suppresses GH release. However, stimulation is dominant over suppression because hypothalamic or hypothalamic-pituitary portal system lesions lead to GH deficiency and not GH excess. GnRH stimulates LH and FSH release. As opposed to the other anterior pituitary hormones, Prl is controlled by suppression by PRIH (dopamine). ACTH, adrenocorticotropic hormone; CRH, corticotropin-releasing hormone; FSH, follicle-stimulating hormone; GH, growth hormone; GHRH, growth-hormone-releasing hormone; GnRH, gonadotropin-releasing hormone; LH, luteinizing hormone; PRIH, prolactin-release inhibiting hormone; Prl, prolactin; SRIH, somatostatin; TRH, thyrotropin-releasing hormone; TSH, thyroid-stimulating hormone.

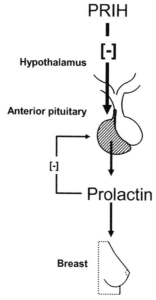

Fig. 2.5 Prolactin secretion is under suppressive control by dopamine (PRIH) that is released by the hypothalamus. Prolactin is secreted by anterior pituitary lactotrophs (mammotrophs). Prolactin can suppress its own release. Prolactin plays a key role in lactation in the postpartum period. PRIH, prolactin-release inhibiting hormone.

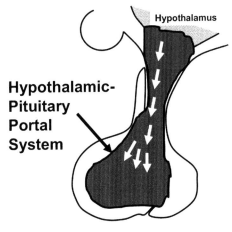

Fig. 2.6 The hypothalamic-pituitary portal system is in gray, with the direction of flow of the portal system depicted in white arrows, bringing hypothalamic releasing and inhibiting hormones to the anterior pituitary.

Measurements

- Prolactin can be measured irrespective of the time of day
  - Morning would be preferred only because most reference intervals are based on fasting measurements in the morning.
- Normally higher in women than in men
  - Rises during pregnancy
  - Remains elevated during the postpartum period
- Measurements can be perturbed by:
  - Macroprolactinemia (i.e., when monomeric prolactin binds to circulating immunoglobulin G creating an antigen-antibody complex [IgG-Prl]); or
  - High-dose hook effect in the prolactin immunoassay.
- Macroprolactin elevates prolactin concentrations and is often asymptomatic.
  - The only way to detect and confirm macroprolactinemia is to remeasure the prolactin after the serum is treated with polyethylene glycol (PEG) to precipitate antigen–antibody complexes with the remeasurement of prolactin in the supernatant.
  - If the prolactin concentration declines by 50% or more, macroprolactinemia is present.
- A true elevation in prolactin can occur coincidentally with macroprolactinemia.

- ○ If prolactin post–PEG treatment is still elevated, true hyperprolactinemia is present and requires clinical evaluation.
- Health care professionals should consider the high-dose hook effect (i.e., a falsely low signal; Fig. 2.7) when a patient has:
  - ○ An anterior pituitary mass but no anterior pituitary hormones levels are elevated; or prolactin is elevated but not proportionate in magnitude to the size of the mass (if the mass is indeed a prolactinoma; Fig. 2.8)

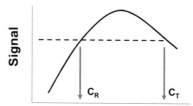

Prolactin concentration

Fig. 2.7 With the high-dose hook effect seen in some immunoassays, the reported concentration (C_R) is much lower than the true concentration (C_T). This occurs due to excessive Prl presence binding both the capture and detection antibody binding sites separately without cross-linking thus producing a falsely low signal.

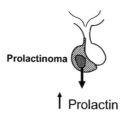

↑ Prolactin

Fig. 2.8 Prolactinomas hypersecrete prolactin. If the prolactin is >200 ng/mL, there is a high likelihood that a prolactinoma is present.

- Diagnosis of a prolactinoma is very important because they are:
  - ○ Usually medically treated with dopamine agonists (e.g., cabergoline); and
  - ○ Not surgically treated unless any one of the following three conditions are met:
    1. The patient does not want to take a long-term oral dopamine agonist.
    2. There is failure to respond to oral dopamine agonists or there is disease progression after an initial response to medical treatment.
    3. Pregnancy is desired in a woman with a microadenoma who cannot tolerate an oral dopamine agonist.
- Radiation therapy is not very effective in treating prolactinomas; therefore, it is not recommended.

Deficiency

- Prolactin deficiency can be a consequence of any destructive lesion involving the anterior pituitary.
- Prolactin deficiency may impair postpartum lactation. Otherwise, prolactin deficiency has no adverse clinical consequences.

Excess

- Prolactin excess can cause galactorrhea in men or women.
- Hyperprolactinemia may impair gonadal function and may cause:
  - In women:
    - Oligomenorrhea;
    - Amenorrhea; or
    - Infertility.
  - In men:
    - Oligospermia; and
    - Erectile dysfunction.
  - The most serious cause of hyperprolactinemia is a prolactin-secreting anterior pituitary tumor (i.e., prolactinoma; Fig. 2.8).
  - Other causes of hyperprolactinemia relate to:
    - Systemic disease (producing stress); and
    - Drugs or dopamine deficiency from hypothalamic disease or disease of the hypothalamic-pituitary portal system (Fig. 2.9).

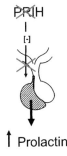

PRIH

↑ Prolactin

Fig. 2.9 Deficiency of PRIH due to hypothalamic disease or disease of the hypothalamic-pituitary portal system can cause hyperprolactinemia. PRIH, prolactin-release inhibiting hormone.

- If the prolactin level is >200 ng/mL, then there is an increased likelihood that a macroprolactinoma is present.
  - Macroprolactinomas are ≥1 cm in diameter, whereas microprolactinomas are <1 cm in diameter.
- Prolactinomas are the most common type of anterior pituitary adenoma.

- Drugs that raise prolactin include:
  - Estrogens;
  - Dopamine receptor blockers;
    - E.g., phenothiazines
  - Dopamine antagonists;
    - E.g., metoclopramide, domperidone
  - Various psychiatric drugs;
    - E.g., haloperidol, risperidone
  - Beta blockers;
  - Calcium channel blockers;
  - Antihistamines; and
  - H2 receptor blockers
    - E.g., cimetidine, ranitidine

Growth hormone

- Also known as somatotropin.
- GH is secreted by anterior pituitary somatotrophs (Fig. 2.10).

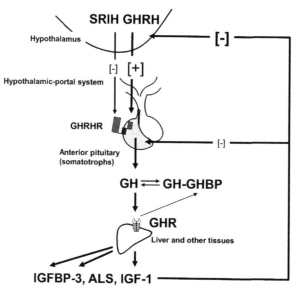

Fig. 2.10 GHRH stimulates the release of GH via binding to its GHRH receptor (GHRHR), whereas SRIH suppresses GH release. Stimulation is dominant over suppression. A portion of GH circulates bound to its binding protein (GHBP), which is the cleaved extracellular domain on the GHR. GH binding to its receptor leads to the secretion of IGF-1, IGFBP-3, and the ALS. IGF-1 feedback centrally is predominantly at the level of the hypothalamus. ALS, acid-labile subunit; GH, growth hormone; GHBP, growth hormone-binding protein; GHR, growth hormone receptor; GHRH, growth-hormone-releasing hormone; GHRHR, growth-hormone- releasing hormone receptor; IGF-1, insulin-like growth factor 1; IGFBP-3, IGF binding protein 3; SRIH, somatostatin.

- The hypothalamus produces GH-releasing hormone (GHRH) and somatotropin release-inhibiting hormone (SRIH) to regulate GH secretion.
  - SRIH = somatostatin
- GHRH and somatostatin reach the anterior pituitary somatotrophs via the hypothalamic-pituitary portal system.
- The predominant control of GH secretion is stimulatory through the action of the GHRH. We know this because hypothalamic disease or disease of hypothalamic-pituitary portal system produces GH deficiency (GHD), not GH excess.
- GH has direct actions on metabolism by elevating free fatty acid levels through lipolysis.
  - This causes insulin resistance, which raises blood glucose.
- In terms of free fatty acids, lipolysis provides an alternative fuel source sparing glucose utilization to sustain the brain and other vital organs.
- With regard to protein metabolism, GH is anabolic.
  - It increases the tissue uptake of amino acids; and
  - Stimulates nitrogen retention and hypoaminoacidemia.
- GH is usually secreted in seven to eight pulses per day.
  - Most of the spikes occurring at night during sleep.
- The indirect growth-promoting effects of GH are the consequence of insulin-like growth factor-I (IGF-1) secretion from GH-responsive tissues.
- Circulating IGF-1 appears to be predominantly the result of hepatic secretion of IGF-1.
  - An older name for IGF-1 is somatomedin C.
- Much of the growth-promoting effects of IGF-1 are local autocrine and paracrine actions (Fig. 2.11).
  - IGF-1 binds to the IGF-1 receptor (IGF1R)
  - IGF-1 can also bind to the insulin receptor (IR). The IGF1R and the IR are highly homologous.
    - Consider an IGF-1R mutation in the setting of short stature, excess IGF-1 is produced by a lack of negative feedback, and may bind the IR (or IGF1R/IR heterodimers) resulting in hypoglycemia.

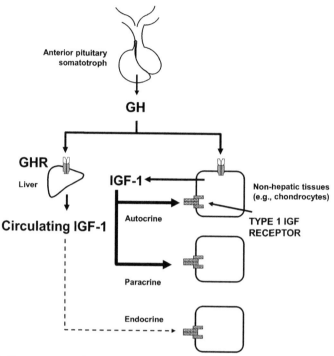

Fig. 2.11 The majority of IGF-1 in the circulation is the product of hepatic IGF-1 secretion. At the tissue level, tissues produce IGF-1 in response to GH. IGF-1 then acts on an autocrine and paracrine basis to produce its effects. GH, growth hormone; GHR, growth hormone receptor; IGF-1, insulin-like growth factor 1.

- GH also stimulates the production of two proteins that circulate together with IGF-1 to form a trimolecular complex:
  - IGF-binding protein-3 (IGFBP-3); and
  - Acid-labile subunit (ALS).
- IGF-1 feeds back centrally to regulate the hypothalamic release of GHRH.
  - Thus, increased IGF-1 reduces GHRH and GH secretion in a negative feedback system.
- Other important factors that regulate IGF-1 levels and the diseases that may lead to growth impairment include (Fig. 2.12):
  - Thyroid hormone—hypothyroidism;
  - Sex steroids—hypogonadism;
  - Chronic disease (may cause increased metabolic demand); and
  - Nutrition—malnutrition.

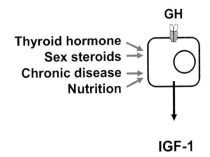

Fig. 2.12 Factors other than growth hormone (GH) regulate IGF-I concentrations. IGF-1, insulin-like growth factor-1.

- GH's downstream hormones are measured in search of GH deficiency (GHD) or GH excess.
- The most significant manifestation of GHD in:
  - Children: Short stature, low growth velocity.
  - Adults: Decreased quality of life, premature cardiovascular disease, osteoporosis, increased fracture risk, reduced muscle mass, increased body fat.
- Genetic defects in the GH-IGF-1 axis impair function and may cause GH insensitivity, bio-inactive GH or IGF-1, or anti-GH antibodies. Genetic variants can occur in the following genes and present with phenotypic characteristics of GHD (growth failure), in addition to other features:
  - *GHR* and *STAT5B*—midface hypoplasia, hypoglycemia (more in *GHR*), pubertal delay (IGF-1 and IGF-BP3 ↓, GH ↑)
  - *PTPN11*—facial dysmorphism, pubertal delay
  - *IGF-1*—facial dysmorphism, deafness, microcephaly, intellectual delay, hyperinsulinism (IGF-1 ↓, GH ↑)
  - *IGFALS*—pubertal delay, hyperinsulinemia (IGF-1 and IGF-BP3 ↓, GH ↑)
  - *IGF1R*—facial dysmorphism, microcephaly (IGF-1 and GH ↑)
  - *GH1* (GH gene)—midface hypoplasia (IGF-1 and IGF-BP3 ↓)
- GH excess is expressed as:
  - Gigantism in children (who have open growth plates) and acromegaly in adults (who have closed growth plates).
  - Both are rare conditions that usually result from a GH-secreting anterior pituitary adenoma.

Measurements

- GH is secreted in a variety of forms.
  - Full-sized GH is composed of 191 amino acids and has a mass of 22 kDa.
  - The 22-kDa form represents 85–90% of circulating GH.
  - The 20-kDa form lacks amino acids 32–46.
    - Measuring the proportion of the total GH that is the 22-kDa form can be important in search of GH doping in sports because recombinant DNA hGH lacks the 20-kDa form of GH and is composed solely of the 22-kDa form.
- GH can dimerize as "big GH."
- GH can also circulate with a GH-binding protein (GHBP) that represents the circulating cleaved N-terminal extracellular domain of the GH receptor (GHR).
  - "Big-big" GH
- Approximately 50% of GH circulates in the free (unbound) state.
- With all of the various forms of circulating GH, measuring GH is a challenging analytical problem.
- The clinical circumstances for measuring GH will be described below.
  - Recall, that GH is secreted in a pulsatile fashion.
  - However, it is accurate to state that random measurements of GH (outside the newborn period) to assess sufficiency or insufficiency are often not informative and cannot be recommended.

IGF-1 and IGFBP-3 measurements

- IGF-1 must be released from its binding protein (IGFBP-3) prior to analysis.
- IGF-1 levels vary by:
  - Age;
  - Sex;
  - Nutritional state; and
  - Degree of sexual maturation of the child.
- IGF-1 can be measured at any time.
  - This is because IGF-1 levels are stable throughout the day.
- Likewise, IGFBP-3 levels vary by (but to a lesser extent than IGF-1):
  - Age;
  - Sex;
  - Nutritional state; and
  - Degree of sexual maturation of the child.

Clinical and laboratory approach to short stature in children

- Short stature in children and adolescents can be defined as height below the third percentile for age and sex.
- Short stature by itself is not a disease as most cases of short stature are familial.
- Short stature in children should be first classified as normal growth velocity or low growth velocity (Fig. 2.13).

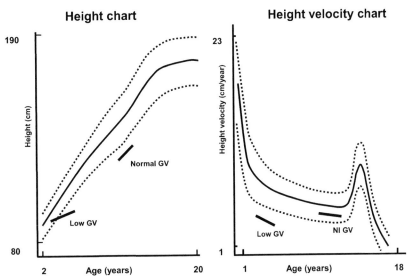

Fig. 2.13 Left: Growth curve for height (cm) versus age in years (actual curves are specific for boys or for girls). The solid line is the average height for age, whereas the dotted lines represent the 97th and the third percentiles. When GV is normal, the child's growth in height will run parallel with the curve. When GV is low, the child's growth in height will fall away from the curve. Right: Height velocity curve (i.e., cm/year of growth) versus age (actual curves are specific for boys or for girls). The solid line is the average height velocity for age, whereas the dotted lines represent the 97th and the third percentiles. When GV is normal, the child's growth in height will run parallel with the curve. When GV is low, the child's growth in height will fall away from the curve. *GV*, growth velocity.

- Normal growth velocity may result from:
  - Familial short stature;
  - Constitutional delay of growth and maturation (also known as "delayed maturation" or "late bloomer"—constitutional delay can also cause a relatively low growth velocity if the child is pre-pubertal and their average peer is pubertal); or

- Primordial short stature (e.g., the child was small at birth and remains small but has a normal growth rate).
- Until age 2, height is measured with the child supine. Beginning after age 2, height is preferably measured standing using a stadiometer for accuracy. Standing, the child places their feet together, looking away from the measuring device, and looks forward. The stadiometer head plate is placed at the crown of the head. Two or three measurements should be taken and averaged.
- Low growth velocity can be serious.
- The causes of low growth velocity are:
  - Malnutrition (failure to thrive);
  - Neglect or psychological abuse;
  - Turner syndrome in girls;
  - Other genetic disorders that involve short stature;
  - Chronic disease; and
  - Endocrine disorders.
- Endocrine disorders causing low growth velocity short stature include:
  - Hypothyroidism (can cause slowed growth or halting of height gain with delayed bone maturation);
  - Glucocorticoid excess (can cause growth plateau);
  - Hypogonadism;
  - Long duration persistently above target glucoses in someone with diabetes; and
  - GHD.
- Hypothyroidism must be excluded in the initial workup for growth failure (decreased growth velocity).
  - This requires TSH and free T4 measurements.
  - TSH alone may be uninformative if TSH or thyrotropin-releasing hormone deficiency are present (e.g., central hypothyroidism).
- Glucocorticoid excess (endogenous or exogenous) is initially evaluated by obtaining the patient's history and performing a physical examination.
  - The details of this workup are explained in the chapter on adrenal disease.
- GHD can present in early infancy with hypoglycemia and/or micropenis in males.
  - It can also present later in life as short stature when the infant's or child's growth velocity is below normal.
- Causes of GHD include:
  - Congenital or structural abnormalities that may or may not cause hypopituitarism.

- o Acquired causes include pituitary/hypothalamic tumors and/or cranial radiation, infiltrative disease, autoimmune hypophysitis, and meningo-encephalitis (the latter three being more common in adults than in children).
- Short stature notwithstanding, children with GHD have increased body fat and an immature facial appearance.
- GHD may result from disease of the:
  - o Hypothalamus;
  - o Hypothalamic-pituitary portal system; or
  - o Anterior pituitary gland.
- If GHD is diagnosed, a search for the cause of GHD is vital.
  - o For example, the underlying cause of GHD may be craniopharyngioma, which would require specific surgical therapy. After therapy for craniopharyngioma, if the infant or child still has GHD, GH replacement therapy should be initiated.
- There are two levels of testing for the diagnosis of GHD.
  1. A low IGF-1 level (not otherwise explained) and/or low IGFBP-3 level.
  2. Because IGF-1 levels may be affected by factors other than GH concentrations, provocative testing may be utilized using a pharmacologic challenge (e.g., arginine, clonidine, glucagon, insulin).
- Fed state lowers GH, whereas the fasted state or exercise raise GH.
- If the GH level rises above the cutoff value for GHD (often 7–10 ng/mL), then GH sufficiency is identified and no further measurements are required.
- Definitive testing for GHD requires that any combination of two stimulatory tests be administered.
  - o This is because only 80% of typical children (i.e., those without growth hormone deficiency) will respond to any one stimulus achieving a sufficient GH level (e.g., usually 7–10 ng/mL).
- If two GH stimuli are administered, then at least 95% of typical children will display a sufficient GH response.
- Priming pre- or peripubertal children with sex steroid (e.g., estradiol or testosterone) increases the peak GH level and may decrease the rate of false positive tests. This is due to the fact that during puberty there is a physiological rise in GH.
- If GHD is diagnosed, then an investigation, if not already performed, for hypothalamic, hypothalamic-pituitary portal system, and pituitary disease should be pursued.

- Although patients may have isolated GHD, multiple anterior pituitary hormone deficiencies are also common.
- Testing adults who have been diagnosed with childhood GHD is required.
  - Not all adults with a history of childhood GHD remain GH deficient throughout adulthood.
- The criterion for the diagnosis of GHD in adults is generally less rigorous than in children.
- If an adult has been diagnosed with a pathogenic genetic variant, irreversible structural lesion, or multiple pituitary hormone deficiencies provocative testing may not be required.
- A stimulated GH level that is lower than 3–5 ng/mL is consistent with GHD in adults.
- If GH is elevated while the IGF-1 level is low, then GH resistance is diagnosed (e.g., Laron syndrome).
  - This results from mutations in the *GHR* or in a signaling pathway (e.g., *STAT5B* loss of function mutations).
- IGF-1 deficiency very rarely results from mutations in the *IGF-1* gene.
- In rare cases, if the GH levels and IGF-1 levels are high, yet the patient has a short stature and low growth velocity, then a loss of function mutation in the IGF-1 receptor (IGF-1R) may be present.
- GHD is treated with daily or weekly subcutaneous injections of recombinant human GH (rhGH).
- Over-the-counter oral amino acid formulations that claim to raise GH secretion in adults (for its supposed anti-aging properties) have no scientific validity in the treatment of children or adults with any known or suspected deficiency of GH.

Excess

- GH excess in children leads to excessive tall stature (gigantism).
- Pituitary adenomas can result in excess secretion of one or more anterior pituitary hormone(s). For example, pituitary adenomas derived of;
  - Somatotrophs presents with GH excess only;
  - Both somatotrophs and corticotrophs can present with clinically apparent GH excess and cortisol excess;
  - Both somatotrophs and lactotrophs can present with symptoms of both GH and prolactin excess.
- Or pituitary adenomas can destroy surrounding normal pituitary tissue causing various pituitary hormone deficiencies in addition to excesses of GH.

- o E.g., GH excess and gonadotropin deficiency, and with the failure of sex steroid production there can be a prolonged period of time when the epiphyses have not fused.
    - This permits continued excessive linear growth late into a person's teenage years or beyond contributing to extreme tall stature in cases of gigantism.
- Although uncommon itself, acromegaly is still much more common than gigantism.
    - o Acromegaly is manifested as enlargement of the:
        - Hands, feet and jaw;
        - Organomegaly;
        - Weight gain;
        - Hyperhidrosis (excessive sweating);
        - Skin tags;
        - Intestinal polyps; and
        - Premature cardiovascular disease.
- GH excess is diagnosed by the finding of an elevated IGF-1 concentration and/or demonstrating that GH is not suppressed (e.g., <2 ng/mL) within 2 h following an oral glucose load (1.75 g/kg to a maximum of 75 g); i.e., an oral glucose tolerance test (OGTT).
- GH excess due to an anterior pituitary adenoma producing GH (a somatotropinoma; Fig. 2.14) is treated surgically.
    - o Other therapeutic modalities include:
        - Pharmacologic GH suppression with octreotide (a somatostatin analog) or bromocriptine; or
        - Pegvisomant, which acts as a GHR antagonist.
- Less commonly, an extra-pituitary somatotropinoma (i.e., a GH-secreting tumor that is outside of the sella), hypothalamic excess of GHRH, or a nonpituitary tumor-secreting GHRH may cause acromegaly.

Posterior pituitary

Physiology

- Vasopressin (antidiuretic hormone; ADH) and oxytocin are the hormonal products of the posterior pituitary gland (Fig. 2.15; also see Fig. 1.22 in the introductory chapter).
- Both hormones are synthesized in magnocellular neurosecretory neurons in the hypothalamus (supraoptic nucleus (SON) and paraventricular nucleus (PVN)).

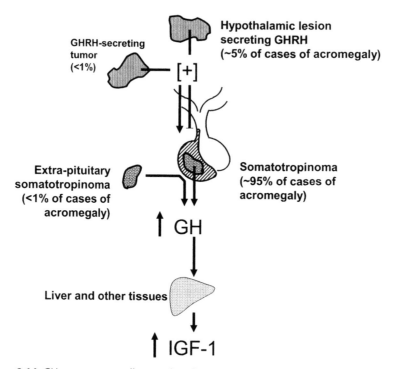

Fig. 2.14 GH excess usually results from a GH secreting anterior pituitary somatotropinoma. Less common causes of GH excess include hypothalamic disorders secreting excess GHRH, nonhypothalamic tumors secreting GHRH (e.g., from the islets of Langerhans), and extra-pituitary somatotropinoma. Elevated GH leads to elevated IGF-1 levels. GH, growth hormone; GHRH, growth-hormone-releasing hormone; IGF-1, insulin-like growth factor 1.

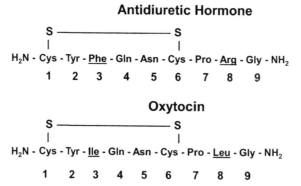

Fig. 2.15 The structures of antidiuretic hormone and oxytocin are illustrated (underlined amino acids are different between structures).

- Axons of these neurons are distributed to the posterior pituitary where hormone storage and secretion occurs.
- Therefore, the posterior pituitary is an extension of the brain (derived from neuroectoderm).

Antidiuretic hormone

- ADH is the preferred term for this posterior pituitary hormone because its primary physiological role is the regulation of free water excretion by the collecting duct of the kidney's nephron. Under normal circumstances, ADH has minimal effect on blood pressure (e.g., "vasopressin" effects). Only when secreted in high concentrations does ADH cause vasoconstriction.
- ADH is a nonapeptide composed of a side chain of three amino acids and a cyclic hexapeptide.
- ADH is secreted in response to increases in plasma osmolality (Fig. 2.16).

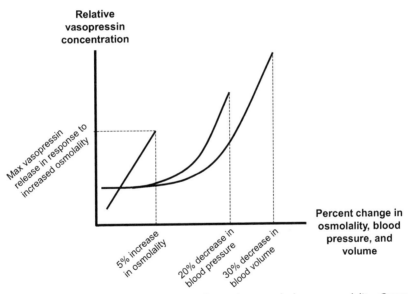

Fig. 2.16 Vasopressin is the most responsive to increased plasma osmolality. Greater declines in blood pressure and blood volume are necessary to elicit vasopressin release.

- Plasma osmolality is sensed by nuclei of the hypothalamus (SON and PVN).
- To lesser degrees, hypotension and hypovolemia release ADH.
  - This latter regulation is via the aortic arch and carotid sinus high-pressure arterial baroreceptors and low-pressure volume receptors located in the atria and pulmonary venous system.

- By binding to the arginine vasopressin receptor-2 (AVPR2) in the nephron's collecting ducts, ADH causes the water channel aquaporin-2 to translocate from a cytoplasmic pool to the plasma membrane of the collecting duct cells adjacent to the lumen of the collecting duct.
- Thus, ADH increases free-water reabsorption from urine in the collecting ducts.
- This increases total body water (reducing plasma osmolality) while increasing the urine osmolality.
- At high concentrations, ADH acts as a vasoconstrictor.

Measurements

- Immunoassays for vasopressin are available in reference laboratories.
- However, in clinical medicine, most disorders of vasopressin, either having excess or deficient vasopressin, are diagnosed using measurements of urine and plasma osmolality and sodium concentration as well as urine volume production over time and body weight (e.g., with ADH deficiency, weight will be lost unless the patient purposefully drinks water to avoid dehydration).
  - Therefore, measurements of ADH are rarely needed.
- However, in cases of partial or unclear diagnosis of diabetes insipidus (DI), ADH levels are available and more recently, the measurement of copeptin.
  - Copeptin is a cleavage product of pre-pro-vasopressin (Fig. 2.17)

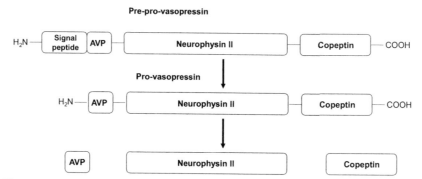

Fig. 2.17 Vasopressin is derived from a pre-pro-hormone (similar to insulin). Neurophysin II (carrier protein) and Copeptin are also stored in the same vesicle as AVP until secretion from the posterior pituitary. Copeptin isolation has led to improved direct testing for diabetes insipidus as AVP is not as reliable to measure. *AVP*, arginine vasopressin.

- The proper interpretation of ADH levels requires that the plasma osmolality be concurrently measured.
  - E.g., if the plasma osmolality is high, then it is physiologic that ADH be near the upper limit of the reference interval.
  - Likewise, if the plasma osmolality is low, then it is physiologic that ADH be near the lower limit of the reference interval.

Hypofunctional disorders
Diabetes insipidus
- Vasopressin deficiency can result from (Fig. 2.18):
  - Developmental, destructive, traumatic, infectious, inflammatory, or neoplastic disorders of the hypothalamus, pituitary stalk (e.g., commonly seen as part of Langerhans cell histiocytosis), or posterior pituitary.

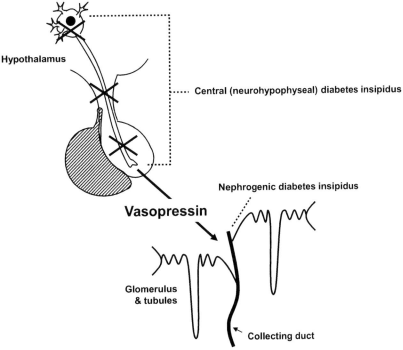

Fig. 2.18 DI results from a failure of vasopressin secretion (central DI) or resistance to the action of vasopressin (nephrogenic DI). DI, diabetes insipidus.

- ADH deficiency causes central diabetes insipidus (DI).
  - Diabetes—"to siphon"; insipidus—"tasteless."

- Polyuria results because of a failure to properly concentrate the urine.
- In contrast to the polyuria seen in diabetes mellitus (mellitus—"sweet"), DI does not result from an osmotic diuresis.
- Polyuria in DI occurs because of decreased free-water recovery from the urine.
- In response to polyuria, a relative state of dehydration occurs, stimulating thirst that initiates increased drinking (e.g., polydipsia).
- In some adults with DI, the urine volume may reach or exceed ~10 L/day.
- DI is diagnosed when polyuria and polydipsia result in hypernatremia and the urine is inadequately concentrated relative to the plasma (and in the absence of hyperglycemia and glucosuria). Individuals may be able to compensate for polyuria with polydipsia, thus restricted access to oral fluids may be required in order for serum hypernatremia to occur and the diagnosis to be made.
- Stated another way, if the plasma osmolality is elevated yet the urine osmolality is low (e.g., the urine is dilute), the kidney is not normally concentrating the urine and DI is possible.
- Although central DI is most often an acquired disorder, congenital forms do exist.
- Mutations in the vasopressin gene can cause an autosomal dominant pattern of inheritance.
- In the autosomal recessive Wolfram syndrome (*WFS1*), DI is one of a variety of problems that include coexistent diabetes mellitus, optic atrophy, deafness, and absence of the corpus callosum.
- Defects in the response of collecting tubules to ADH cause nephrogenic DI where there is resistance to ADH (Fig. 2.18).
- The classic test in search of DI is the water deprivation test (Fig. 2.19).
  - Typically, the patient is admitted to the hospital (sometimes after an overnight fast) and the patient is maintained NPO (nil per os; nothing by mouth). At baseline, plasma (or serum) sodium, and urine and serum osmolalities are measured.
  - As the fast proceeds, urine volume is carefully recorded and the laboratory work is repeated approximately every 4 h along with the patient's body weight and vital signs.
  - If the patient's body weight declines by 3% or more, then the frequency of monitoring should be increased to every 2 h.
- If DI is present, there is no significant reduction in the urine volume over time, the urine remains dilute and the plasma osmolality and sodium rises.

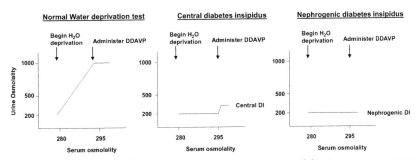

Fig. 2.19 *Left:* With normal vasopressin secretion, urine osmolality increases as serum osmolality increases. DDAVP does not increase the urine osmolality further because the urine will be maximally concentrated via the action of endogenous vasopressin. *Middle:* In central DI, the urine does not concentrate with water deprivation; however, the urine osmolality will increase after administration of DDAVP. *Right:* In nephrogenic DI, there is no response to DDAVP. There are partial forms of central and nephrogenic DI that will have findings intermediate between normal and complete DI. DDAVP, 1-deamino-8-D-arginine vasopressin; DI, diabetes insipidus.

- With DI, the urine osmolality remains low despite increased plasma osmolality. What would normally happen in the absence of DI is that the urine osmolality (e.g., >600–1000 mOsm/kg) will exceed the plasma osmolality as the urine volume decreases with time. Typical criteria to support the diagnosis of DI include (cutoff values vary slightly by reference):
  - Hypernatremia (Na >145 mmol/L)
  - Plasma osmolality >300 mOsm/kg
  - Urine osmolality <300 mOsm/kg
  - Urine sodium <30 mEq/L
  - Urine specific gravity <1.010
  - Urine output >4 mL/kg/h (>5 mL/kg/h in infants)
- Once DI is diagnosed, 1-desamino-8-D-arginine vasopressin (DDAVP, also known as desmopressin) may be administered (Fig. 2.20).
- Although patients with central DI will concentrate their urine in response to the administration of DDAVP, urine osmolality does not rise in response to DDAVP in patients with nephrogenic DI.
- Thus, the response of the urine osmolality to DDAVP can be used as a diagnostic test to distinguish central versus nephrogenic DI.
- Alternatively, ADH (or copeptin) could be measured as being inappropriately low in central DI and elevated in nephrogenic DI (see above).
- Nephrogenic DI may be congenital or acquired.

Antidiuretic Hormone (aka, arginine vasopressin)

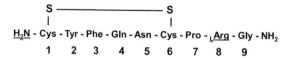

DDAVP (aka, 1-desamino-8-D-arginine vasopressin)

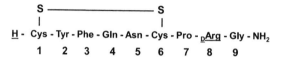

Fig. 2.20 The structures of antidiuretic hormone and the synthetic replacement, DDAVP, which are enantiomers, where the same compounds have an opposite 3-D shape, indicated by an ʟ (levo) or ᴅ (dextro) (underlined amino acids are different between structures).

- o E.g., from urinary tract obstruction, hypercalcemia, hypokalemia, use of certain drugs (amphotericin B, lithium, and the antibiotic demeclocycline)
- Congenital nephrogenic DI may be inherited as an X-linked recessive disorder from mutations in the *AVPR2* gene or in an autosomal dominant or autosomal recessive pattern from mutations in aquaporin-2 (Fig. 2.21).
- Other causes of polyuria and polydipsia include defective function of the renal tubules (the proximal and the distal convoluted tubules are also necessary to properly concentrate the urine), and primary polydipsia (increased thirst due to psychiatric disease or medication).
- Osmotic diuresis is excluded from the differential diagnosis of DI.
  - o This is because the urine osmolality is high in an osmotic diuresis, which is not the case with DI.
- In patients with DI, if thirst is impaired (e.g., by hypothalamic disease or injury) or access to water is restricted, then hypernatremia may occur. Management becomes very challenging in the absence of an intact thirst mechanism.

Hyperfunctional disorders
- ADH excess can result from:
  - o Stress (e.g., cardiopulmonary disease, pain, nausea)
  - o Central nervous system disease (e.g., meningitis, encephalitis); or
  - o Drugs (e.g., vincristine, cyclophosphamide, chlorpropamide, sulfonylureas, nonsteroidal anti-inflammatories, opiates, tricyclic antidepressants, haloperidol).

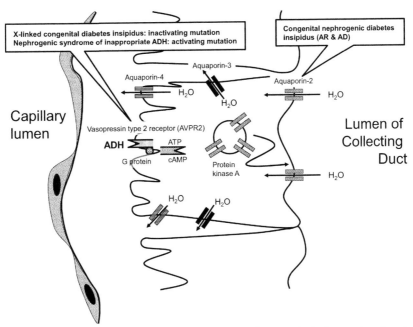

Fig. 2.21 Congenital nephrogenic DI can be inherited as an X-linked recessive disorder from mutations in AVPR2 or in an autosomal dominant or recessive pattern from mutations in aquaporin-2. An activating mutation of AVPR2 causes a nephrogenic form of SIADH. AD, autosomal dominant; ADH; antidiuretic hormone; AR, autosomal recessive; ATP, adenosine triphosphate; AVPR2, arginine vasopressin receptor 2; cAMP, cyclic adenosine monophosphate; DI, diabetes insipidus; SIADH, syndrome of inappropriate antidiuretic hormone secretion.

- ADH excess may be physiologic (e.g., in the setting of blood loss) or may cause the syndrome of inappropriate antidiuretic hormone (SIADH).
  - Reminder: vasopressin = antidiuretic hormone.
- In SIADH there is excessive ("inappropriate") reabsorption of water from the collecting ducts.
- This increases total body water and urine volume is reduced and excessively concentrated in spite of hypo–osmolar plasma.
- This free water retention can cause hyponatremia.
- SIADH is usually treated by restricting a patient's intake of free water.
  - It is important to consider all sources of fluid intake (including IV medications, for example, as often this volume can be substantial).
- Sodium can also be increased by the administration of hypertonic saline (3% sodium chloride = 513 mEq/L of NaCl) if hyponatremic seizures develop. Furosemide is not often recommended as a treatment in

children. Similarly, newer agents, V2-receptor antagonists (conivaptan and tolvaptan) have only been studied thus far in adults.
- If the serum sodium is too rapidly corrected, central pontine myelinolysis with permanent neurologic deficits may result.
  - Therefore, care and patience are important in the treatment of SIADH and depend on the time frame over which hyponatremia initially developed.
  - Typically, when treating hyponatremia, the increase in the plasma sodium concentration should not exceed 4–5 mEq/L per 24 h.

Oxytocin

- Like ADH, oxytocin is a nonapeptide composed of a cyclic hexapeptide and a side chain with three amino acids.
- Oxytocin is released in response to suckling when the breast has been hormonally prepared for lactation during the postpartum period.
- Contraction of smooth muscle cells in the breast propels milk toward the nipple, a phenomenon termed "milk letdown."
- Oxytocin also causes constriction of uterine smooth muscle.
- When it is synthetically prepared, oxytocin can be administered to initiate or strengthen uterine contractions during labor, and it also can be administered after delivery of the newborn and placenta to cause uterine contraction to reduce blood loss.
- There are no known diseases of oxytocin deficiency or excess; therefore, there is no clinical indication to measure oxytocin.

Hypopituitarism and molecular testing

- Hypopituitarism or the presence of multiple pituitary hormone deficiencies, can be:
  - Congenital or
  - Acquired
- Congenital hypopituitarism
  - Presentation in the neonatal period can include:
    - Persistent hypoglycemia in infancy (GH deficiency and/or central adrenal insufficiency)
    - Persistent neonatal jaundice
      1. Indirect hyperbilirubinemia (central hypothyroidism, central adrenal insufficiency)
      2. Direct hyperbilirubinemia (central adrenal insufficiency, GH deficiency)

- Small phallus size in XY males (GH deficiency, LH/FSH deficiency)
- Polyuria/hypernatremia (ADH deficiency)
- Midline defects: cleft lip and/or palate, single central incisor, holoprosencephaly, optic nerve hypoplasia, absent or hypoplastic septum pellucidum and/or corpus callosum
- Once one pituitary hormone defect is found in infancy, assessment for other pituitary hormone deficiencies is prudent.
- Disorders: Optic nerve hypoplasia (ONH; formerly known as septo-optic dysplasia)
  o More prevalent in infants born to mothers of younger age (± maternal substance abuse)
  o *HESX1* variants are seen in ONH; however, genetic confirmation is rarely found.
  o Visual defects and GH deficiency are common abnormalities; although, multiple pituitary hormone deficiencies (MPHD) are also common.
- In addition to *HESX1*, other transcription factors are essential in the formation of the pituitary (Fig. 2.22).
  o Molecular testing can be considered for those with MPHD.
  o Variants in *PROP1* are the most common genetic cause of MPHD and may result in combinations of pituitary hormone deficiencies (GH, TSH, Prl, evolving LH/FSH, ACTH deficiencies).
  o PIT1 (GH, TSH, Prl deficiencies)
  o LHX3 (GH, TSH, Prl, LH/FSH ± ACTH deficiencies; associated feature: rigid cervical spine)
  o LHX4 (variable deficiencies from isolated GHD to panhypopituitarism; associated feature: cerebellar abnormalities)
  o TPIT (Congenital isolated adrenocorticotropin deficiency—impaired *POMC* transcription resulting in low to no ACTH, rarely responds to CRH administration; associated features: FTT, severe hypoglycemia, jaundice)
  o OTX2 (variable deficiencies; ocular malformation)
- Acquired causes of hypopituitarism may include,
  o Pituitary or hypothalamic tumor or surgery for removal of such a tumor
  o Traumatic brain injury affecting the pituitary
  o Radiation therapy to the head or neck
  o Autoimmune hypophysitis
  o Meningitis, encephalitis
  o Sarcoidosis, Langerhans cell histiocytosis

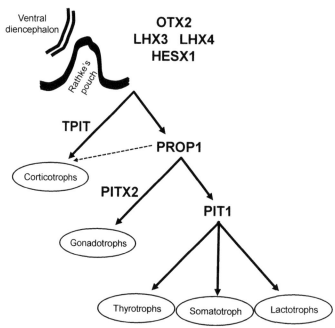

Fig. 2.22 Several transcription factors are involved along the development pathway that leads to the mature cells of the anterior pituitary as demonstrated in this simplified diagram. OTX2, Orthodenticle homeobox 2; LHX3, LIM-homeobox 3; LHX4, LIM-homeobox 4; HESX1, Homeobox gene expressed in stem cells 1; TPIT, T-box transcription factor, pituitary; PROP1, Homeobox protein prophet of Pit-1; PITX2, Paired-like homeodomain transcription factor 2; PIT1, pituitary-specific transcription factor 1.

Conclusion

- The anterior and posterior pituitary glands are embryologically, structurally, and functionally distinct.
- With the exception of oxytocin, deficiencies and excesses causing clinical disease are associated with all of the products of the anterior and posterior pituitary glands.
- For most hormones, random measurements are not informative.
- In cases of potential anterior pituitary hormone excess, suppressive testing is usually required to diagnose a true excess of the hormone.
- In cases of potential anterior pituitary hormone deficiency, stimulatory testing is usually required to diagnose a true deficiency of the hormone.
- Some hormones can be assessed in random plasma measurements such as prolactin.
- Congenital hypopituitarism can present with a variable phenotype and pituitary hormone deficiencies.

Suggested reading

Development and microscopic anatomy of the pituitary gland—Endotext—NCBI Bookshelf (nih.gov).

de Oliveira R, Longo Schweizer J, Ribeiro-Oliveira Jr A, Bidlingmaier M. Growth hormone: isoforms, clinical aspects and assays interference. Clin Diabetes Endocrinol 2018;28(4):18. https://doi.org/10.1186/s40842-018-0068-1. PMID: 30181896. PMCID: PMC6114276.

Fang Q, George AS, Brinkmeier ML, Mortensen AH, Gergics P, Cheung LYM, Daly AZ, Ajmal A, Millán MIP, Bilge Ozel A, Kitzman JO, Mills RE, Li JZ, Camper SA. Genetics of combined pituitary hormone deficiency: roadmap into the genome era. Endocr Rev 2016;37(6):636–75. https://doi.org/10.1210/er.2016-1101.

Hiers PS, Winter WE. Biochemistry of growth. In: Dietzen DJ, Wong ECC, Bennett MJ, Haymond S, editors. Biochemical and molecular basis of pediatric disease. 5th ed; 2021. p. 327–78.

Mason A, Malik A, Ginglen JG. Hypertonic fluids. In: StatPearls. Treasure Island, FL: StatPearls Publishing; 2023. Available from: https://www.ncbi.nlm.nih.gov/books/NBK542194/.

Rivkees SA, Dunbar N, Wilson TA. The management of central diabetes insipidus in infancy: desmopressin, low renal solute load formula, thiazide diuretics. J Pediatr Endocrinol Metab 2007;20(4):459–69. https://doi.org/10.1515/jpem.2007.20.4.459. PMID: 17550208.

Saugy M, Robinson N, Saudan C, Baume N, Avois L, Mangin P. Human growth hormone doping in sport. Br J Sports Med 2006;40(Suppl. 1):i35–9. https://doi.org/10.1136/bjsm.2006.027573. PMID: 16799101. PMCID: PMC2657499.

Savage MO, Hwa V, David A, Rosenfeld RG, Metherell LA. Genetic defects in the growth hormone-IGF-I axis causing growth hormone insensitivity and impaired linear growth. Front Endocrinol (Lausanne) 2011;2:95. https://doi.org/10.3389/fendo.2011.00095. PMID: 22654835. PMCID: PMC3356141.

CHAPTER 3

Thyroid gland

Physiology

- Hormonal products of the thyroid gland (Fig. 3.1) include:
  - Thyroxine (T4, or 3,5,3′,5′ tetraiodothyronine) and
  - Triiodothyronine (T3, or 3,5,3′ triiodothyronine).
- Thyroid hormone exists as free (biologically active) and bound (inactive) fractions.
- Free thyroid hormone is biologically made up of free T4 (FT4) and free T3 (FT3). FT4 and FT3 are measured individually. Note: In most clinical circumstances, total T3 can be measured instead of FT3.
- In the circulation, most T4 (99.97%) and T3 (99.7%) are bound to thyroxine-binding proteins.
- T4 has one-tenth the biologic activity of T3.
  - Of the total amount of T3 in the circulation, there is proportionally 10 times as much unbound T3 (0.3%) as unbound T4 (0.03%).
- T4 can be considered a prohormone for T3 because 80% of T3 is generated by monodeiodination of T4 to T3 in peripheral tissues (e.g., the liver).
- The conversion of T4 to T3 is influenced by the state of health of the individual.
  - For example, acute, severe illness or chronic illness results in decreased conversion of T4 to T3 and increased levels of reverse T3 (rT3, or 3,3′,5′ triiodothyronine; Fig. 3.1).
- This state describes the sick euthyroid syndrome (also known as nonthyroidal illness [NTI]), which will be discussed below.
- The most important thyroxine-binding protein is thyroxine-binding globulin (TBG).
- Elevated TBG is caused by:
  - Estrogen;
  - Pregnancy;
  - Acute liver disease;
  - Phenothiazines; and
  - Hereditary excess.

Quick Guide to Endocrinology
https://doi.org/10.1016/B978-0-443-14135-5.00002-8

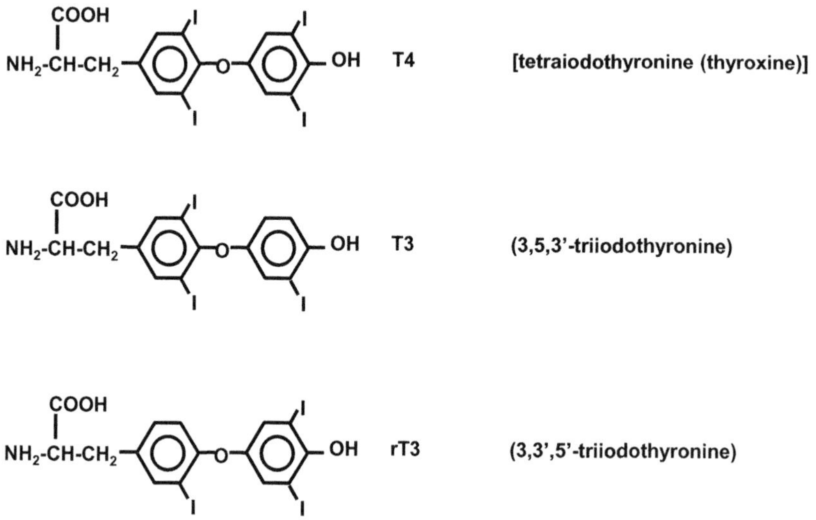

Fig. 3.1 Structural formulas for T4, T3, and rT3.

- Low TBG results from:
  - Androgens;
  - Glucocorticoids;
  - Excess of growth hormone;
  - Chronic liver disease;
  - Protein loss (e.g., nephrosis, protein-losing enteropathies); and
  - Hereditary deficiency.
- rT3 is not biologically active. There are few clinical circumstances where the measurement of rT3 is clinically informative.
- All thyroid hormones are metabolized by peripheral monodeiodination (Fig. 3.2).

Thyroid hormone

Actions

- Thyroid hormone:
  - Increases the basal metabolic rate;
  - Is vital for normal growth and central nervous system development in infants and children; and
  - Stimulates the metabolism of various drugs and hormones.
- Thyroid hormone enters cells via monocarboxylate transporters (e.g., monocarboxylate transporter 8).

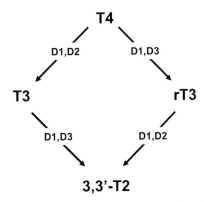

Fig. 3.2 Deiodinases (D1, D2, and D3) convert T4 to either T3 or rT3. Subsequent deiodinations of T3 and rT3 produce various isomers of diiodothyronine (T2), including the 3,3'-T2 isomer (not shown are the 3,5-T2 and 3',5'-T2 isomers). Deiodinases vary by location (D1-liver and kidney; D2-heart, muscle, CNS, fat, thyroid, and pituitary; D3-fetus, placenta, and brain [except in pituitary]). Infantile hepatic hemangiomas overproduce D3 resulting in rapid degradation of T4 and T3 (i.e., consumptive hypothyroidism).

- o In target cells (e.g., the pituitary thyrotrophs and hepatocytes), T4 is converted to T3.
- The thyroid hormone receptors (TRs; TR alpha and TR beta) serve as transcription factors to regulate gene expression.
  - o Loss-of-function mutations in TR beta produce thyroid hormone resistance and a possible hypothyroid state.
  - o A TR alpha mutation has been described that produces hypothyroidism with only borderline abnormal thyroid function tests.

Synthesis

- Thyroid follicular cells concentrate iodide through active transport via the sodium/iodide symporter (NIS) on the basal surface of the cell (Fig. 3.3).
  - o This is under control of thyroid-stimulating hormone (TSH, also called thyrotropin).
- After iodide has entered the cytoplasm of the thyroid follicular cell, iodide is pumped into the colloid via pendrin (encoded by the *SLC26A4* gene) that is located on the apical pole of the thyroid follicular cell.
- The thyroid follicular cell synthesizes thyroglobulin (Tg), which is also controlled by TSH.
- Tg is secreted into the colloid.

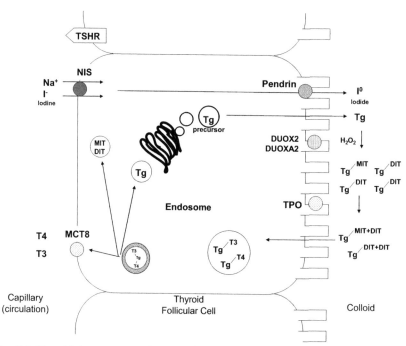

Fig. 3.3 Thyroid hormone synthesis is depicted. Refer to the text for details. DIT, diiodothyronine; MIT, monoiodothyronine; Tg = thyroglobulin; TSHR = TSH receptor; NIS = sodium-iodine symporter; DUOX2/DUOXA2 = dual oxidase 2/dual oxidase maturation factor 2; TPO, thyroid peroxidase; MCT8 = Monocarboxylate transporter 8.

- Tyrosines that are part of Tg are iodinated by the action of thyroperoxidase (TPO) on the apical border by converting iodide (I^-) to iodine (I^0).
- Tg iodination produces monoiodothyronine (MIT) and diiodothyronine (DIT).
- Via the coupling activity of TPO within Tg, T4 and T3 are formed.
- Under the influence of TSH, the colloidal Tg is pinocytosed by the apical membrane of the thyroid follicular cell.
- After this pinocytotic vesicle is fused with an endosome, Tg is digested, thus releasing T4 and T3.
- T4 and T3 exit the thyroid follicular cell into the adjacent interstitial fluid and diffuse into the circulation to be bound by:
  ○ TBG;
  ○ Thyroxine-binding prealbumin (TBPA, also known as transthyretin); and
  ○ Albumin.

- TBPA carries very little T3.
- Within the thyroid follicular cell, released MIT and DIT are deiodinated by iodothyronine deiodinase to recycle iodine within the gland that is then available for new thyroid hormone synthesis.
- With increased stimulation of the gland via the TSH receptor, T3 synthesis and release increases to a greater extent than T4 synthesis and release. However, the majority of the time T4 is the dominant hormone synthesized and released from the thyroid gland.
- rT3 is formed from T4 by an alpha (inner) ring deiodination (D1, D3).

Regulation

- The hypothalamus secretes thyrotropin-releasing hormone (TRH) in a tonic pattern in response to decreased negative feedback from reduced thyroid hormone concentrations (Fig. 3.4).

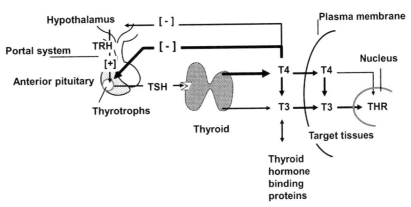

Fig. 3.4 Regulation of thyroid hormone secretion. Refer to the text for details. THR = thyroid hormone receptor.

- TRH travels to the anterior pituitary via the hypothalamic-pituitary portal system binding to TRH receptors on the anterior pituitary thyrotrophs which release TSH.
- TSH is an alpha-beta glycoprotein hormone.
- Luteinizing hormone (LH), follicle-stimulating hormone (FSH), human chorionic gonadotropin (hCG), and TSH share a common alpha subunit.
  o Each of these glycoprotein hormones has a unique beta-subunit (Fig. 3.5).

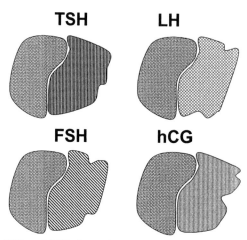

Fig. 3.5 TSH, LH, FSH, and hCG share the same alpha subunit but have unique beta subunits.

- TRH is necessary for the proper glycosylation of the TSH subunits to achieve full biologic activity.
  - TSH enters the systemic circulation to bind to TSH receptors expressed on thyroid follicular cells and stimulates increased secretion of T4 and T3.
- Thyroid hormones negatively exert feedback on the hypothalamus, and, more importantly, on the anterior pituitary thyrotrophs.
  - Negative feedback at the level of the pituitary is predominantly due to FT4. Within the pituitary, by deiodination T4 is converted to T3 to provide a negative signal for TSH release.
    - The relationship between TSH and FT4 is an inverse log-linear relationship (Fig. 3.6).

Measurements

- Thyroid-related hormones that can be measured are (note: Tg can also be measured):
  - TSH;
  - Total T4;
  - FT4;
  - Total T3;
  - FT3; and
  - rT3.
    - "Total" T4 and T3 immunoassays measure free and bound thyroid hormones.

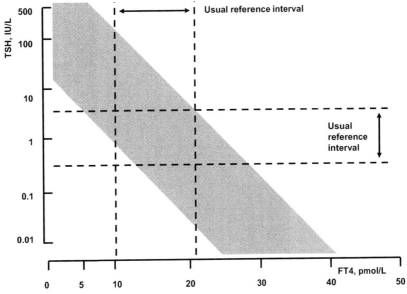

Fig. 3.6 Inverse log-linear relationship between TSH and FT4. FT4, free T4; TSH, thyroid-stimulating hormone.

- The gold standard for free thyroid hormone assays is the dialysis equilibrium (DE) assay.
  - Most laboratories use a second generation, two-step immunoassay to measure free thyroid hormone levels.
- FT4 is the preferred measurement rather than total T4. This is because FT4 is less affected by the levels of thyroid-hormone binding proteins, which may have a large effect on total T4.
  - Historically, total T4 measurements were used along with a T3 resin uptake (T3RU, T-uptake) to estimate the free T4.
  - T3RU is an indirect measure of TBG binding capacity.
    - Briefly, radioactively labeled T3 is added to the patient's serum sample where it binds to open binding sites on TBG (Fig. 3.7). The remaining labeled T3 is taken up the resin (i.e., T3 resin uptake). If euthyroid, in the setting of declining TBG levels, fewer open binding sites would be present and more labeled T3 would bind to the resin (i.e., T3RU rises). Conversely, if euthyroid, in the setting of rising TBG levels, more open binding sites are available for labeled T3 to bind to with less labeled T3 taken up by the resin (i.e., T3RU declines).

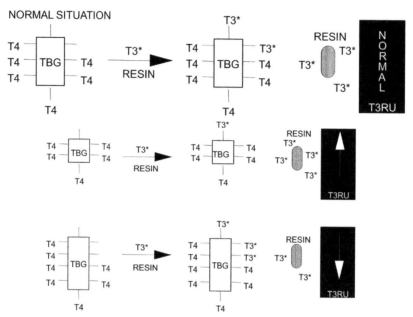

Fig. 3.7 Top panel: In the T3 resin uptake test, in vitro radioactively labeled T3 binds to open binding sites on TBG. The unbound T3 then binds to the resin (albumin). Middle panel: Assuming that the patient is euthyroid, if TBG levels are reduced, there are fewer open binding sites on TBG and more T3 binds to the resin. Bottom panel: Assuming that the patient is euthyroid, if TBG levels are increased, there are more open binding sites on TBG and less T3 binds to the resin.

- T4 is carried by TBG (predominantly), prealbumin (also known as transthyretin), and albumin, whereas T3 is carried by TBG and albumin (Fig. 3.8).

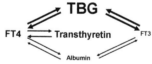

Fig. 3.8 T4 is carried on thyroxine-binding globulin (TBG), transthyretin (a.k.a., thyroxine-binding prealbumin), and albumin. T3 is carried on TBG and albumin. The bound hormones are in equilibrium with the free hormones (FT4 = free thyroxine and FT3 = free triiodothyronine).

- TBG has the highest affinity for T4 and T3 but TBG has the lowest capacity.
- Albumin has the highest capacity for T4 and T3 but it has the lowest affinity.
- Another historical test to assess causes of thyroid gland dysfunction is the perchlorate discharge test.
  - In this test, administered radioactive iodine is taken up by the thyroid and given time to be incorporated into the organification process.

Then, perchlorate is given which will displace, or "discharge," any non–organified iodide from the thyroid. If a large amount of the radio-active iodine is discharged rapidly the test is abnormal and a sign of potential dyshormonogenesis.

- T3 is not a first-line measurement of thyroid function and total T3 is more accurately measured than FT3. Total T3 measurements when T3 must be measured are usually sufficient, although other experts may prefer FT3.
- The current TSH double-antibody (sandwich, or non-competitive) immunoassays measure to a lower limit of detection (LLD) of approximately 0.01 µIU/mL (3rd generation TSH assay) and 0.001 µIU/mL (4th generation TSH assay). At this level:
  - For robust assays, the coefficient of variation should be no greater than 20%.
    - Chemiluminescence or electrochemiluminescence is used.
- Second generation TSH assays had a LLD of approximately 0.1 µIU/mL. Such assays should not be used.
  - These assays could determine whether TSH was low but not the degree of suppression (e.g., whether TSH is just slightly low or depressed to the very low levels seen in Graves disease [GD]).
- Because most TSH assays are double-antibody assays, human anti-mouse antibodies (HAMA), if present, may falsely increase TSH (Fig. 3.9).

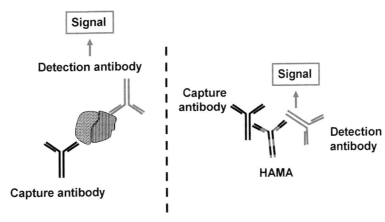

Fig. 3.9 On the left, a typical double-antibody (sandwich-type) immunoassay is depicted in which the capture antibody "collects" the analyte (TSH in this case) and the detection antibody indicates the concentration of the analyte by the signal that it generates. On the right, human anti-mouse antibodies (HAMA) can crosslink the capture antibody and the detection antibody falsely indicating that analyte is present.

Thyroid-related autoantibodies

- Measurements of the various thyroid-related autoantibodies are very helpful in assessing the cause of thyroid dysfunction.
- Autoantibodies against thyroid peroxidase (TPOA) and/or thyroglobulin (TGA) do not distinguish Hashimoto thyroiditis (HT) or atrophic thyroiditis (AT; see discussion below) from GD.
  - ○ The presence of either of these autoantibodies indicates that a patient has some form of thyroid autoimmunity, most often euthyroid HT
- Autoantibodies directed against the TSH receptor (e.g., thyroid-stimulating hormone receptor antibodies [TRAbs]) can be agonists (e.g., thyroid-stimulating immunoglobulins [TSIs]) or antagonists that cause AT.
- TRAbs can be assayed as TSIs or thyrotropin-binding inhibitory immunoglobulins (TBIIs).
- In the TSI assays, serum (with suppressed TSH levels) may stimulate thyroid follicular cells in vitro (Fig. 3.10).

Thyroid stimulating immunoglobulins (TSIs)

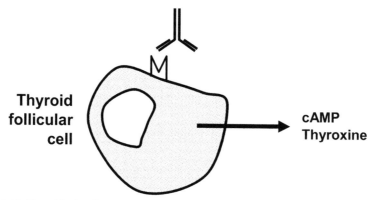

Fig. 3.10 Thyroid-stimulating immunoglobulins (TSIs) are detected by the capacity of a patient's serum to stimulate thyroid follicular cells in vitro to produce cyclic AMP (cAMP) or thyroxine (T4).

- In the TBII assay, immunoglobulin in serum competes with labeled TSH for binding to TSH receptors in vitro (Fig. 3.11).
  - ○ The TBII test does not distinguish agonist versus antagonistic TRAbs.
  - ○ The TRAb and TBII assay names are not well standardized across laboratories, while TSI is a separate, easy-to-find bioassay.

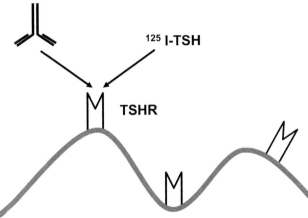

Fig. 3.11 Thyrotropin-binding inhibitory immunoglobulins (TBIIs) are measured in vitro as TSH receptor autoantibodies that compete against labeled-TSH for binding to TSH receptors (TSHR). (Note: the TSHRs are present on isolated membranes).

- The distributions of thyroid autoantibodies in various autoimmune thyroid diseases are depicted in Table 3.1.

Table 3.1 Thyroid autoantibody tests.

Autoantibody	Target autoantigen	AITD distribution
TPOA	TPO	HT, AT, GD
TGA	Tg	HT, AT, GD
TSI[a]	TSH-R (agonist)	GD
TBII[a]	TSH-R: blocks TSH binding to TSH-R[b]	AT, GD

[a]TSI or TBII are uncommon in HT.
[b]TBII positivity does not indicate whether TRAb stimulates or blocks the TSH-R.
AITD, autoimmune thyroid disease; AT, atrophic thyroiditis; GD, Graves disease; HT, Hashimoto thyroiditis; TBII, thyrotropin-binding inhibitory immunoglobulin; Tg, thyroglobulin; TGA, thyroglobulin autoantibody; TPO, thyroid peroxidase; TPOA, thyroid peroxidase autoantibody; TRAb, thyroid-stimulating hormone receptor antibody; TSH-R, thyroid-stimulating hormone receptor; TSI, thyroid-stimulating immunoglobulin.

Thyroglobulin
- Thyroglobulin (Tg) is detected in the plasma of normal individuals.
- Measurements of Tg can be used to evaluate:
  o Whether the patient's own gland is active. Tg measurements are employed as a tumor marker in cases of differentiated thyroid cancer after surgical removal (however, baseline Tg should be measured preoperatively to ensure that the tumor does produce Tg before it is used a tumor marker).
  o In cases of congenital hypothyroidism, if Tg is not detected in the plasma, then the diagnosis of thyroid aplasia is supported.

- If patients who are euthyroid take excessive doses of thyroxine (e.g., factitious hyperthyroidism), then the Tg level can be depressed or unmeasurable.
- Tg is measured by immunoassay.
  - Its concentrations are proportionate to thyroid gland mass and activity.
- TGA interferes with the Tg assay.
  - If TGA is positive, the Tg level is not interpretable unless the Tg is measured by competitive immunoassay (e.g., RIA) or by mass spectroscopy.

External influences on thyroid function or laboratory measurement

- Chronic illness may alter thyroid function (see the discussion about sick euthyroid syndrome below).
- Iodine excess or deficiency can alter thyroid function.
- Iodine can be present in:
  - High concentrations in various radiologic contrast media;
  - Certain drugs (e.g., amiodarone); and
  - Topical solutions used to clean the skin or peritoneal dialysis catheters (e.g., povidone-iodine).
- Chronic iodine deficiency causes endemic goiter and even hypothyroidism.
- Similarly, termed the "Wolff-Chaikoff effect," iodine excess in the short term can suppress thyroid function (Fig. 3.12) in iodine sufficient geographic areas.
  - Thus, high-dose iodine can be used preoperatively to reduce the vascularity of the thyroid gland prior to thyroidectomy for patients with Graves disease. This can reduce surgical blood loss.
  - The thyroid normally recovers (or "escapes") from such suppression after approximately 10 days of high-dose iodine administration.
- In a patient who is iodine deficient but euthyroid, replenishing iodine may allow the expression of hyperthyroidism.
  - Known as the "Jod-Basedow" phenomenon (Fig. 3.12).
  - Iodine deficiency remains prevalent throughout the world (Fig. 3.13).
- L-Dopa, dopamine, glucocorticoids, somatostatin, somatostatin analogs, and rexinoids (retinoid X receptor agonists) may reduce TSH secretion.
  - Potentially leads to a decline in thyroid hormone levels
- Lithium is widely used to treat bipolar disorder.
  - May cause hypothyroidism; lithium (which is concentrated in the thyroid gland) inhibits iodine uptake by the thyroid.
  - Cases of hyperthyroidism have also been described

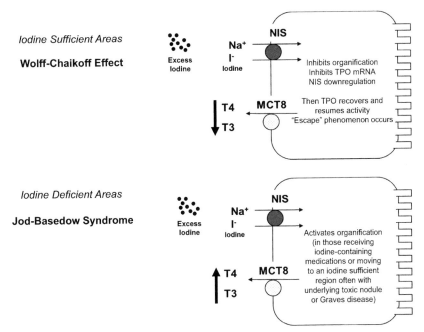

Fig. 3.12 Excess iodine exposure or ingestion can lead to contrasting phenomenon based on level of iodine sufficiency in the region resulting in reduced thyroid hormone secretion or excess. NIS = sodium-iodine symporter; TPO, thyroid peroxidase; MCT8 = Monocarboxylate transporter 8.

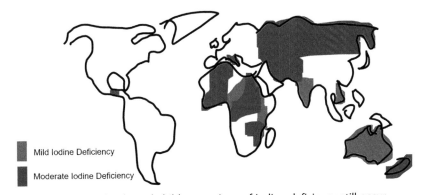

Fig. 3.13 Among school-aged children, regions of iodine deficiency still occur.

- Drugs that impair the conversion of T4 to T3:
  - Propylthiouracil (PTU);
  - Amiodarone;
  - Beta blockers;

- ○ Glucocorticoids; and
- ○ Contrast agents.
- Drugs that displace thyroid hormone from TBG can decrease total T4 and total T3.
  - ○ Free thyroid hormone levels may remain normal or may even increase.
  - ○ Includes furosemide, nonsteroidal anti-inflammatory agents, salicylates, carbamazepine, phenytoin, and heparin.
- Elevated metabolism of thyroid hormone can lower T4 and T3.
  - ○ Rifampicin, phenytoin, phenobarbital, carbamazepine.
- Supplements or drugs may also impair thyroid hormone absorption from the gut in the treatment of hypothyroidism.
  - ○ E.g., sodium polystyrene sulfonate, iron, calcium, aluminum hydroxide, soybean preparations, cholestyramine, colestipol.
- Various cytokines used to treat viral infectious diseases (e.g., hepatitis) may also alter thyroid function. For routine cases of hepatitis C, cytokines are not used in its treatment.
- Interferon alpha may cause autoimmune or nonautoimmune thyroiditis.
  - ○ May lead to hypothyroidism
  - ○ Transient hyperthyroidism from an intense destructive phase of thyroiditis is possible (analogous to Hashitoxicosis)
- Prolonged administration of nitroprusside may cause hypothyroidism when isothiocyanate competes with iodide (I^-) for thyroid gland uptake.
- Therapeutic radiation for cancers, such as Hodgkin lymphoma, that include the neck may induce hypothyroidism.
- It is possible for hypothyroidism or hyperthyroidism to follow bone marrow transplantation in children.
- Drugs and other treatments can induce actual functional changes in the thyroid gland; however, the presence of laboratory interferences that have no direct effect on thyroid function but may dramatically affect clinical decision making are important to review.
  - ○ Biotin supplementation interferences are discussed below.
- Other hormonal changes can affect immunoassay measurements without changing physiological thyroid function.
  - ○ In the case of obesity, elevated leptin (released from adipocytes), stimulates TRH and TSH release from the hypothalamus and pituitary, respectively (Fig. 3.14).
  - ○ In the setting of obesity, the mild elevations in TSH level preferentially stimulate the release of T3 (not T4) from the thyroid.

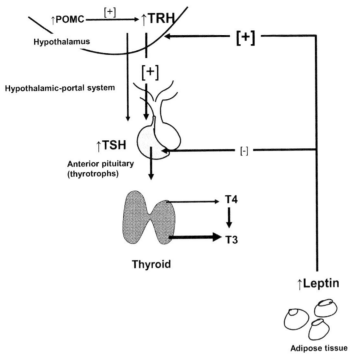

Fig. 3.14 Elevated leptin levels, correlated to adiposity, stimulates hypothalamic production of TSH directly and via TRH stimulation. Mild elevations in TSH can be mistaken for hypothyroidism but studies of children with and without obesity indicate that this is not true hypothyroidism.

- Use of biotin supplementation to "strengthen hair and nails" has increased dramatically. Beyond those with a congenital or acquired cause of biotin deficiency, there is limited evidence to support biotin supplementation. Recommended daily allowance (RDA) of biotin is 30 µg which is typically ingested in our foods. Over-the-counter supplements contain up to 100,000 µg (>3000 times more than the RDA)
  - Biotin (water soluble vitamin B7) is used in a variety of immunoassays due to the high affinity bond between the small biotin molecule and the large streptavidin protein (which also conjugates to a reporter molecule for measurement).
  - High-dose biotin supplementation, therefore, can affect many hormone assays (Table 3.2). Biotin interferences occur with competitive and non-competitive immunoassays (refer to Chapter 1, Figs. 1.26–1.28).

Table 3.2 Examples of high-dose biotin supplement interference on several endocrine hormone immunoassays.

	Assay	Interference
Competitive	FT4, FT3	Falsely high
	Testosterone	Falsely high
	Estradiol	Falsely high
	DHEAS	Falsely high
	Cortisol	Falsely high
Non-competitive	TSH	Falsely low
	Thyroglobulin	Falsely low
	PTH	Falsely low
	LH	Falsely low
	FSH	Falsely low

- Competitive immunoassays: excess free biotin binds to the antibody in place of the "competitor." Low levels of the competitor are then measured as if the "competitor" was "knocked off" the antibody by the patient's analyte. Therefore, due to the inverse relationship between the analyte of interest and the assay output, this results in a falsely high signal.
- Non-competitive immunoassays: excess free biotin prevents the binding of the biotin-labeled detection antibody with the streptavidin. This leads to less fluorescence, for example, and a falsely low signal.

Thyroid disorders

- Disorders of thyroid function may involve increased size of the gland (i.e., goiter), thyroid nodules (including thyroid cancer), and/or dysfunction, including hypothyroidism, hyperthyroidism, as well as compensatory states such as that seen in sick euthyroid syndrome.

Goiter and nodules

- Goiters are either:
  - Asymmetric; or
  - Symmetric (e.g., diffuse) (Fig. 3.15).
- An asymmetric goiter may result from a:
  - Large thyroid nodule;
  - Hypoplasia of a lobe; or

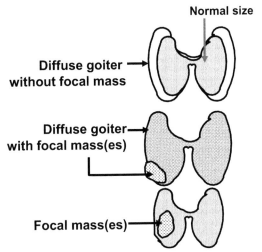

Fig. 3.15 Enlargement of the thyroid gland can be diffuse (top panel); a diffusely enlarged gland can also include a focal mass or masses (middle panel); or the enlargement can be strictly focal, such as a thyroid nodule in the absence of diffuse goiter (bottom panel).

- o Hypoplasia of a portion of a lobe of the thyroid.
- A diffuse goiter and a nodule (or nodules) within the thyroid gland can coexist.
  - o Nodules detectable by palpation are generally ≥2 cm in diameter.
- The vast majority of thyroid nodules are benign.
  - o Benign nodules may be caused by hyperplasia, a cyst, an intrathyroidal lymph node, or a bacterial abscess (e.g., acute thyroiditis).
- Thyroid nodules occur less frequently in children compared to adults (<5% vs 30% via ultrasound detection).
- The risk of a thyroid nodule in children being cancerous is higher than in adults
- The risk of metastasis and recurrence is higher in pediatric thyroid cancer but the overall prognosis is still good.
- Goiter and thyroid nodules must be distinguished from other neck masses such as:
  - o Adenoma, hyperplasia, or carcinoma of the parathyroid glands;
  - o Neoplastic, infectious, or autoimmune lymphadenopathy;
  - o Aneurysms of arteries or veins;
  - o Soft-tissue neoplasms (e.g., laryngeal carcinoma);
  - o Malformations (e.g., thyroglossal duct cyst); and

- ○ Neck muscle traumatic damage.
- These distinctions are made predominantly by physical examination and imaging studies unless:
  - ○ Cancer is present that is metastatic to the cervical lymph nodes; or
  - ○ Hematopoietic malignancy of the lymph nodes (e.g., lymphoma) is diagnosed where biopsy and flow cytometry may provide vital information.
- The differential diagnoses of diffuse goiter includes:
  - ○ Hashimoto thyroiditis (HT);
  - ○ Graves disease (GD);
  - ○ Colloid goiter;
  - ○ Iodine deficiency;
  - ○ Inborn errors in thyroid hormone synthesis; and
  - ○ Goiter of pregnancy.
- Except for cases of colloid goiter, a goiter in hypothyroid HT, GD, iodine deficiency, inborn errors, and goiter of pregnancy results from stimulation of the TSH receptor.
- In cases of HT with normal TSH values (euthyroid HT), a goiter may result from infiltration of the gland by lymphocytes accompanied by chronic inflammation (i.e., chronic lymphocytic thyroiditis).
- In hypothyroid HT, iodine deficiency, and inborn errors, the TSH receptor is stimulated by high levels of TSH.
- In GD, the TSH receptor is stimulated by TSIs.
- In goiter of pregnancy, the TSH receptor is stimulated by high levels of hCG.

Colloid and multinodular goiters
- Colloid goiters do not cause thyroid dysfunction.
- Idiopathic enlargement of the thyroid follicles may lead to a diffuse goiter.
- Although biopsy will establish the diagnosis of a colloid goiter, there are no laboratory tests for a colloid goiter. Thyroid autoantibodies are absent.
- Over time, a colloid goiter may evolve into a multinodular goiter in which some areas of the thyroid gland continue to hypertrophy (forming palpable nodules), whereas other regions of the gland undergo atrophy.
- If a nodule(s) becomes autonomously hyperactive, then hyperthyroidism may result.
  - ○ The result is a toxic nodule or toxic multinodular goiter (called Plummer disease).
    - ▪ "Toxic" here refers to the development of hyperthyroidism.

Hypothyroidism

- Hypothyroidism essentially is a deficiency of thyroid hormone accompanied by clinical findings of hypothyroidism (Table 3.3).

Table 3.3 Characteristic findings in hypothyroidism.

Symptoms seen in children, adolescents, and adults	
Tiredness	Constipation
Cold intolerance	Dry hair/skin
Growth failure	Oligomenorrhea/ amenorrhea
Slow mentation	Bradycardia
Low pulse pressure	Myxedema
Congestive heart failure	Coma
Hypercholesterolemia	Elevated creatine kinase
Hyporeflexia (specifically, delayed relaxation phase)	Delayed bone age

Symptoms seen in infants/neonates if untreated	
Poor tone	Macrosomia
Poor feeding	Large fontanel
Macroglossia	Prolonged jaundice
Umbilical hernia	Hoarse cry

- Hypothyroidism can be classified as:
  - Primary (thyroid gland failure);
  - Secondary (TSH deficiency); or
  - Tertiary (TRH deficiency).
  - Secondary and tertiary hypothyroidism can collectively be termed "central" hypothyroidism.
- Causes are outlined in Table 3.4.
- Pituitary disease causing TSH deficiency and secondary hypothyroidism is uncommon and accounts for only 1% of acquired cases of hypothyroidism.
  - *Congenital hypothyroidism*: Cretinism is the clinical description of the adverse consequences of hypothyroidism in the newborn; however, the term cretinism is an archaic term and is not used.
  - The preferred term is congenital hypothyroidism.
  - In the United States, the advent of the Newborn Screening Program wholly has markedly reduced the incidence of severe congenital hypothyroidism.

Table 3.4 Causes of hypothyroidism.

Primary hypothyroidism (thyroid gland failure)

Inflammatory or infectious causes

Autoimmune thyroid disease
- Hashimoto thyroiditis
- Atrophic thyroiditis
- Late-stage Graves disease (a "burned out" thyroid gland)
- Postpartum thyroiditis
- Viral or bacterial thyroiditis

Anatomic causes of primary hypothyroidism

Developmental disorders involving the thyroid gland
- Congenital hypothyroidism: aplasia, hypoplasia
- Ectopic thyroid: lingual thyroid, thyroglossal duct cyst
- Surgical removal of the thyroid gland (post-thyroidectomy)

Iodine, drugs, radiation, and dietary goitrogens

Iodine excess or deficiency

Thioamides (e.g., propylthiouracil, methimazole)

Lithium

Nitroprusside

Amiodarone

Biologics (e.g., interferon, interleukin-2)

Radiation-induced hypothyroidism

Inborn errors in thyroid hormone biosynthesis, transport, or uptake into cells (dyshormonogenesis)

Na^+/iodide pump dysfunction

Inadequate organification/iodination—thyroid peroxidase dysfunction

Defective thyroglobulin

Deiodinase deficiency

Pendred syndrome (hypothyroidism and deafness)

MCT8 deficiency (Allan-Herndon-Dudley syndrome)

Secondary hypothyroidism[a]

Pituitary disease with TSH deficiency (see Chapter 2 for etiologies)

Tertiary hypothyroidism[a]

Hypothalamic disease with TRH deficiency (see Chapter 2 for etiologies)

---

[a]Also referred to as central hypothyroidism.

TRH, thyrotropin-releasing hormone; TSH, thyroid-stimulating hormone.

- Congenital hypothyroidism from thyroid gland aplasia or hypoplasia (1:2500–3500 live births) is much more common than congenital hypothyroidism of central origin (e.g., TRH or TSH deficiency).
  - Congenital central hypothyroidism: Frequency of 1 in nearly 100,000 newborns

- Molecular testing could reveal rare genetic causes of central hypothyroidism and can be considered in familial cases and the absence of apparent pituitary lesions:
  - Inactivating mutation in TRH receptor
  - TSH beta-subunit mutation
  - Pituitary transcription factors leading to multiple hormone deficiencies (e.g., HESX1, LHX3, LHX4, PROP1, PIT1)
- Screening for congenital hypothyroidism in North America is performed by measuring total T4 on dried blood spots (with or without TSH). In Europe, TSH is measured for newborn screening (which could miss the rare congenital central hypothyroidism cases).
- Causes of congenital hypothyroidism and their frequency are
  - Hypoplasia, aplasia, or ectopy of the thyroid gland—85%
  - Defect in thyroid hormone synthesis or transport (dyshormonogenesis) often with a goiter (can be detected in utero) due to lack of negative feedback on TSH stimulation of the thyroid—10–15%
  - Thyrotropin (TSH) resistance (TSH receptor mutation)
  - Transient causes of congenital hypothyroidism:
    - Excess iodine
    - Iodine deficiency
    - Maternal anti-thyroid drugs (e.g., methimazole)
    - Maternal TSH receptor antibody (TBII)
    - Congenital hepatic hemangiomas (increased deiodinase type 3; D3) leading to a consumptive hypothyroidism
- Drugs/substances that cross the placenta from mother to fetus:
  - Methimazole
  - PTU
  - Thyroid autoantibodies
  - TRH
  - T4
- Hypothyroxinemia of prematurity is caused by immaturity of the hypothalamic-pituitary-thyroid axis and is a transient process where T4 and TSH in the low normal reference range is detected.
  - The T4 level improves over time as the baby reaches term (i.e., corrected gestational age of 40 weeks).
  - Treatment, in general, is not recommended for hypothyroxinemia of prematurity, owing to concerns of poorer neurologic outcomes in infants who have been treated.

Diagnosis and treatment of primary hypothyroidism

- The measurement of TSH distinguishes primary hypothyroidism (TSH is elevated) from central hypothyroidism (TSH is inappropriately normal or low). In some cases of central hypothyroidism, TSH may be marginally elevated when TSH has reduced bioactivity but normal immunoreactivity.
  - Reduced bioactivity results from abnormal glycosylation induced by TRH deficiency or pituitary disease.
  - TRH testing is no longer used to distinguish primary hypothyroidism from secondary or tertiary hypothyroidism.
- If a patient is believed to have normal pituitary and hypothalamic function, then screening for primary hypothyroidism should begin with a TSH measurement (often with a FT4 simultaneously if the level of concern is high).
  - If TSH is within the reference interval, primary hypothyroidism is excluded.
- The goals of Na-L-thyroxine treatment are to eliminate symptoms of hypothyroidism and to maintain TSH and FT4 levels within the age-appropriate reference intervals. For congenital hypothyroidism, clinicians often will pursue treatment to raise FT4 into the upper half of the reference interval. Na-L-thyroxine replacement is required for life in congenital hypothyroidism.
- The most common cause of primary hypothyroidism in areas of the world with iodine sufficiency is Hashimoto thyroiditis.

Hashimoto thyroiditis (HT)

- HT is a form of autoimmune thyroid disease in which glandular destruction progresses over time.
- The condition is diagnosed upon finding:
  - Positive thyroid autoantibodies (TPOA, TGA, or both) with or without a goiter;
  - With or without biochemical hypothyroidism.
- Therefore, thyroid autoantibodies should be measured to determine the cause of hypothyroidism when primary hypothyroidism is biochemically and clinically diagnosed.
- TSI and TBII are typically negative in cases of HT and should not be ordered.
- A less common form of thyroiditis termed atrophic thyroiditis (AT) results from antagonistic TSH receptor autoantibodies that block the action of TSH causing hypothyroidism (see discussion above).

- o In AT, a goiter will not develop. Typically, TBIIs are positive but TSIs are negative in AT.
- o Antagonistic TSH receptor autoantibodies that cross the placenta can induce a state of temporary primary hypothyroidism in the fetus and subsequent newborn. With subsequent metabolism of the antagonistic TSH receptor autoantibodies, normal thyroid function can return. The differential diagnosis is congenital aplasia or hypoplasia of the thyroid gland.
- HT may also be referred to as chronic lymphocytic thyroiditis because there is a heavy lymphocytic infiltration into the gland.
  - o Lymph node-like follicles can be histologically observed in the thyroid in cases of HT and inflammation is also often displayed by ultrasound imaging.
- The mechanism of glandular destruction is predominantly cell-mediated autoimmunity (despite the presence of thyroid autoantibodies).
- Patients with HT may initially experience a euthyroid goiter. Later in the natural history of HT, a goiter and hypothyroidism can develop.
- In long-standing HT, the thyroid gland may be reduced in size as a result of progressive destruction.
  - o Chronic inflammation may cause fibrosis of the gland.
- Occasionally, patients with HT may experience an accelerated phase of thyroid gland destruction with subsequently excessive and unregulated release of preformed thyroid hormone from cell-mediated destruction that causes transient hyperthyroidism.
  - o Termed "Hashitoxicosis" or "Toximoto" disease
- HT affects women (and girls) more often than men (and boys).
  - o The frequency of HT increases with advancing age.
- In families, HT often appears to be inherited as an autosomal dominant trait, although no single gene has been identified as a causative factor.
  - o HT and GD are frequently found in different members of the same family.
- Pernicious anemia is frequency coexistent with HT or GD.
- Autoimmune thyroid disease affects approximately 25% of girls with type 1 diabetes mellitus (T1DM) and half as many boys with T1DM.
  - o Clinical thyroid disease is experienced in 50% of children with autoimmune thyroid disease and T1DM.
- Of these affected children, 80% have HT, whereas 20% have GD.
- Autoimmune disease, especially HT and GD, are more common in the setting of abnormal chromosome number (e.g., Trisomy 21).

Hyperthyroidism

- Hyperthyroidism is diagnosed by the finding of an elevated total T3 and/ or FT4 (FT3 levels are less reliable) accompanied by clinical findings of hyperthyroidism (Table 3.5).

Table 3.5 Characteristic findings in hyperthyroidism.

Nervousness	Erratic behavior
Emotional lability	Restlessness
Sleeplessness	Trouble concentrating
Smooth, shiny hair and skin	Weight loss
Excessive sweating	Heat intolerance
Menstrual irregularities	Diarrhea or frequent bowel movements
Tachycardia	Atrial arrhythmias
Systolic murmurs	Increased pulse pressure
Vigorous pulse	Warm, damp skin
Soft texture of skin	Tremor
Increased reflexes	Hypocholesterolemia

Additional findings seen in neonates with hyperthyroidism:

Jaundice	Irritability/hyperexcitability
Frontal bossing	Poor feeding
Craniosynostosis	Small fontanelle

- Hyperthyroidism can be classified as:
  - Primary (thyroid gland hyperactivity);
  - Secondary (TSH excess); or
  - Tertiary (TRH excess).
    - Secondary and tertiary hyperthyroidism can be termed central hyperthyroidism.
- Central hyperthyroidism is very rare and may be caused by:
  - TSH-secreting anterior pituitary adenoma (1–2 cases per 1 million); or
  - Selective pituitary resistance to thyroid hormone with normal peripheral (non-pituitary) response to thyroid hormone.
- Rarely, ovarian teratomas, ovarian serous or mucinous cystadenomas hypersecrete thyroid hormone, resulting in hyperthyroidism (called struma ovarii).
  - Struma ovarii falls outside the primary versus central hyperthyroidism classification because the thyroid gland is not the source of the excess thyroxine.
  - Struma ovarii causes a paraneoplastic syndrome similar to the production of adrenocorticotropic hormone by an oat cell carcinoma of the lung or parathyroid hormone-related peptide (PTHrP) synthesis by a tumor producing hypercalcemia.

- Causes of primary hyperthyroidism are outlined in Table 3.6.
  - Most cases result from stimulation of the TSH receptor by TSIs.
  - When present in very high concentrations, hCG can stimulate the TSH receptor.
    - Therefore, hCG-induced hyperthyroidism results from high levels of hCG activating the TSH receptor (Fig. 3.16).

Table 3.6 Causes of primary hyperthyroidism.

Inflammatory or infectious disorders
Autoimmune thyroid disease
- Graves disease
- Hashitoxicosis
- Postpartum thyroiditis
Thyroid destruction from viral or bacterial thyroiditis
Gain-of-function mutation in the TSH-R
Toxic nodule ("hot" nodule)
Toxic multinodular goiter (Plummer disease)
Toxic follicular adenoma
Familial (germline gain-of-function mutation in the TSH-R)
Hyperstimulation of the TSH-R via high levels of hCG
Gestational transient thyrotoxicosis
TSH-R sensitivity to hCG
hCG-secreting tumors
Other disorders
Iodine-induced hyperthyroidism

hCG, human chorionic gonadotropin; TSH-R, thyroid-stimulating hormone receptor.

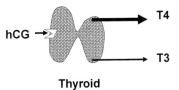

Thyroid

Fig. 3.16 Goiter (and even hyperfunction) can result from hCG binding to the TSH receptor of the thyroid follicular cells.

- If a thyroid nodule overproduces thyroid hormone, then primary hyperthyroidism can develop.
  - Hyperactive nodules may exhibit gain-of-function mutations in the TSH receptor so the receptor is active without binding its ligand (i.e., TSH).
  - Such hyperactive nodules have been described as "toxic nodules" or "hot nodules."

- ○ When multiple nodules are hyperactive in the setting of multinodular goiter, this is termed "toxic multinodular goiter," which is also known as Plummer disease.
- ○ In adults, toxic multinodular goiter is the second-leading cause of primary hyperthyroidism following GD (see discussion below).
- ○ When a nodule is encapsulated, the pathology is considered to be a toxic follicular adenoma.
- ○ Only rarely are thyroid cancers functional.
- ○ Thyroid scintigraphy visualizes toxic nodules as excessively concentrating isotope (^{123}I or technetium-99m) leading to the descriptive term "hot nodule."
- ○ With suppression of endogenous TSH secretion below the lower limit of detection because of hyperthyroidism, other areas of the thyroid gland display reduced isotope uptake and are described as being "cold."
- • Iodine-induced hyperthyroidism is believed to occur as follows:
  - ○ An otherwise hyperthyroid patient maintains a euthyroid state only because of concurrent iodine deficiency.
  - ○ Replenishment of iodine supplies sufficient iodine to synthesize excess thyroid hormone which then unmasks the patient's true hyperthyroidism.
- • Ingestion of excess thyroid hormone (thyrotoxicosis factitia) can produce hyperthyroidism.
  - ○ Strictly speaking, this is not a type of primary hyperthyroidism because the source of thyroid hormone is exogenous.
  - ○ Findings suggestive of thyrotoxicosis factitia include:
    - ■ Hyperthyroidism in the absence of goiter or nodules;
    - ■ Low levels of thyroglobulin (because TSH and the patient's own thyroid gland are suppressed); and
    - ■ Reduced uptake of radioactive iodine (^{123}I).
    - ■ If due to T3 ingestion (whereas TSH will be suppressed and T3 [or FT3] will be elevated), FT4 may be low because the thyroid gland is not stimulated by TSH.
- • Commonly, the only other condition that produces hyperthyroidism in the setting of reduced radioactive iodine uptake is Hashitoxicosis in which thyroid hormone is released from a damaged gland (see the discussion of HT above).

Thyroid storm
- • The most serious complications of hyperthyroidism encompass high output congestive heart failure and thyroid storm.

- Thyroid storm is a clinical diagnosis.
  - No one set of thyroid function test results indicate that a patient with hyperthyroidism is (or is not) experiencing storm.
- With "storm" there is a life-threatening state of extreme hyperthyroidism accompanied by:
  - Hypermetabolism;
  - Fever;
  - Sweating;
  - Poor feeding;
  - Weight loss;
  - Fatigue;
  - Cardiorespiratory distress (e.g., tachycardia, heart failure, hypertension, respiratory distress);
  - Gastrointestinal problems (e.g., nausea, vomiting, jaundice, abdominal pain, diarrhea); and
  - Neurologic disorders (e.g., anxiety, altered behavior, seizures, coma).
- Death from heart failure is possible.

Diagnosis and treatment of primary hyperthyroidism
- TSH measurement distinguishes primary hyperthyroidism (TSH is suppressed) from central hyperthyroidism (TSH is inappropriately normal or elevated)
  - If the patient has normal pituitary and hypothalamic function:
    - Screening for primary hyperthyroidism begins with a TSH measurement.
      - If the TSH is within the reference interval:
        - Primary hyperthyroidism is excluded ("ruled out").
      - If the TSH is suppressed below the reference interval, primary hyperthyroidism is present.
        - If the FT4 is within the reference interval and TSH is repeatedly suppressed:
          - Measure T3 (or FT3).
- Patients with suppressed TSH, normal FT4, and elevated T3 (or FT3) are described as having "T3 toxicosis" which is less common than having elevated T4 or T4 + T3 levels.
  - Can represent an early stage in the evolution of primary hyperthyroidism or may occur in the setting of iodine deficiency.
    - Similarly, an individual with a repeatedly suppressed TSH and symptoms of hyperthyroidism could be early in the disease process.

- However, as an important reminder, a TSH value slightly below the reference range without symptoms of hyperthyroidism may be normal. The laboratory-provided reference range was developed to confidently detect a normal value for 95% of the population encompassing 2 standard deviations above and below the mean. Thus, up to 2.5% of the population may have a TSH value below this reference range (and up to 2.5% above the reference range) (Fig. 3.17).

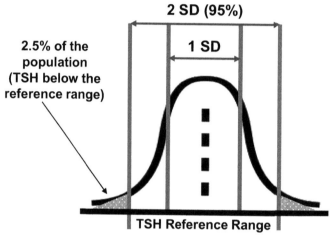

Fig. 3.17 For the majority of laboratory tests, the "normal" or reference range is defined as values falling within 2 standard deviations (SDs) of the mean, where 9% of individual's values will be found. However, this does not account for 5% of individuals who could have a laboratory value above or below this range and still be "normal" (i.e., without disease).

- ○ It is reasonable to assume that iodine deficiency in the setting of hyperthyroidism may produce T3 toxicosis because T3 synthesis requires 25% less iodine than T4 synthesis.
- Treatments for primary hyperthyroidism are outlined in Table 3.7.
- Medical therapy will induce remission in approximately 30% of treated patients.
- Thyroidectomy should be performed by surgeons who have done at least 30 similar surgeries per year. Nevertheless, even in the best of circumstances, surgical complications may be possible.
- There is concern that radioactive iodine treatment can lead to malignancies, and there may also be an increased risk for cardiovascular disease with its use.

Table 3.7 Treatments for primary hyperthyroidism.

Type	Agents/ mechanisms	Examples	Comments
Medical	Drugs that block thyroid hormone synthesis	Propylthiouracil	Potential serious hepatotoxicity (black box warning) Also blocks peripheral conversion T4 to T3
		Methimazole	When used in pregnancy, possible teratogenicity[a]
Surgical	Thyroidectomy		Complications include parathyroidectomy and laryngeal nerve paralysis
Irradiation	Thyroid destruction	^{131}I	Concern about future malignancy (controversial)[b]

[a]Choanal atresia, dysmorphic facies, aplasia cutis, gastrointestinal anomalies—thus avoid methimazole in the first trimester of pregnancy.
[b]Radioactive iodine (RAI) therapy is contraindicated in the setting of a very large gland due to decreased efficacy and also contraindicated in the setting of thyroid eye disease because RAI can be associated with increased thyroid antigen release resulting in increased TSH receptor antibodies that can target orbital cells.

Graves disease

- Graves disease (GD) is a form of autoimmune thyroid disease in which humoral autoimmunity is predominant.
- Pathophysiologically, agonist autoantibodies directed against the TSH receptor cause primary hyperthyroidism (Fig. 3.18). The agonist autoantibodies are termed TSIs (thyroid-stimulating immunoglobulins).
  - TSIs are a form of TRAb (TSH receptor autoantibodies)
  - This is one of the few conditions where the autoantibodies are involved in the disease pathophysiology (e.g., TSIs in GD, acetylcholine receptor antibodies in myasthenia gravis) as opposed to a marker of cellular immunity (e.g., HT, type 1 diabetes autoantibodies)

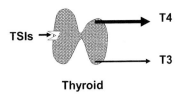

Thyroid

Fig. 3.18 Hyperfunction of the thyroid gland results from TSI binding to the TSH receptor of the thyroid follicular cells. TSI, thyroid-stimulating immunoglobulin.

- By contrast in AT, there are antagonist autoantibodies that block the TSH receptor, thus causing hypothyroidism and thyroid atrophy.
- Classic clinical findings in GD include:
  - Goiter and hyperthyroidism;
  - Exophthalmos; and
  - Pretibial myxedema (more common in adults).
- Exophthalmos can rarely be observed in cases of HT or in the absence of functional thyroid abnormalities.
  - Thyroid eye disease, or Graves orbitopathy, is the most common extra-thyroidal manifestation of Graves disease.
  - Need to consider and exclude other causes of exophthalmos such as retro-orbital tumor.
- The cause of pretibial myxedema is a perplexing clinical finding because pretibial myxedema can be found in GD or HT with hypothyroidism
- Following longstanding Graves hyperthyroidism not treated by surgery or radiation, thyroid gland destruction may occur and evolve into hypothyroidism.
- GD is more common in women than in men.
  - Similar to HT and AT
- GD diagnosis is made by the findings of:
  - Clinical and biochemical hyperthyroidism (e.g., suppressed TSH and elevated T3 [or FT3] with or without an elevated T4 [or FT4] level); plus
  - Thyroid autoantibody positivity (TPOA or, less commonly, TGA).
- TSI or TBII measurements, which are often send-out tests, are not required to diagnose the condition unless TPOA and TGA are negative.
- Like HT and AT, pernicious anemia is common in patients with GD and positivity for gastric parietal cell autoantibodies predicts the development of vitamin B12 deficiency and achlorhydria or hypochlorhydria with impaired iron absorption.
- Propylthiouracil (PTU) can produce liver failure and has fallen out of favor except for in the first trimester of pregnancy.

Neonatal Graves disease

- Maternal hyperthyroidism can produce signs and symptoms of:
  - Hyperthyroidism (e.g., congestive heart failure);
  - Preeclampsia; or
  - Premature labor.

- Potential adverse effects of methimazole on the fetus include:
  - Facial dysmorphism;
  - Choanal atresia
  - Cutis aplasia; and
  - Gastrointestinal anomalies such as esophageal atresia with or without concurrent tracheo-esophageal fistula.
  - When a woman who is pregnant uses either PTU or methimazole, these drugs can cross the placenta and cause fetal hypothyroidism.
- TSIs and antagonist TRAbs may cross the placenta to influence fetal and neonatal thyroid dysfunction.
  - TSIs may cause transient hyperthyroidism or, rarely, thyroid storm in the newborn.
- Fetal hyperthyroidism may manifest as:
  - Tachycardia;
  - Intrauterine growth retardation;
  - Hyperactivity; and
  - May even induce abortion.
- Hyperthyroidism in newborns may cause different symptoms than older children (see Table 3.4) and neonatal Graves disease carries up to a 20% risk of mortality.
- The diagnosis of neonatal Graves disease is made by TRAb positivity plus abnormal thyroid function tests (TFTs) in the baby which are typically obtained on days 3–5 and 10–14 in the setting of maternal or neonatal TRAb positivity. Due to challenges obtaining serum samples in this age, the TRAb assay can be run on a cord blood sample. Mothers with a history of Graves disease should be screened in the third trimester for maternal TRAb positivity. If the mother is negative for TRAb, the risk of the baby developing neonatal Graves disease is negligible.
  - Close monitoring for symptoms is also vital during this time with a low threshold for treatment with MMI.
- Antagonistic TRAbs produce nonpermanent hypothyroidism (elevated TSH and low FT4) or hyperthyrotropinemia (elevated TSH with a normal FT4).
- Maternal TSI levels predict the likelihood of hyperthyroidism in the fetus and newborn (i.e., higher TSI titers translate into higher risk).
- On a separate note, a large goiter from any cause may result in asphyxia immediately following birth.
  - Therefore, if a goiter is noted in the setting of possible fetal hypothyroidism, then intrauterine administration of Na-L-thyroxine should be considered to reduce the size of the goiter to reduce airway obstruction.

Sick euthyroid syndrome

- During times of acute severe or chronic illness, thyroid function is altered, which is termed the sick euthyroid syndrome or nonthyroidal illness.
- Typically, there is reduced conversion of T4 to T3, and T3 (and FT3) levels decline.
- rT3 levels rise because of the impaired degradation of rT3.
- This decline in T3 may be interpreted as adaptive. With decreased caloric intake or decreased oxygen delivery to the issues, lower T3 levels will reduce calorie and energy requirements of the body, which would be beneficial.
- With longer-standing illness, TSH may decrease and can be followed later by a decline in T4 (and FT4) concentrations.
- Sick euthyroid syndrome with decreased TSH may pose a diagnostic challenge in differentiating this condition from central hypothyroidism. In such a case, if the patient manifests clinical findings of hypothyroidism, then a trial of Na-L-thyroxine would not be unreasonable.
- After managing the underlying illness, sick euthyroid should resolve without therapy.
- The diagnosis of sick euthyroid syndrome is based on the clinical setting of acute severe or chronic illness that is usually accompanied by variable TSH and FT4 with a reduced T3 (or FT3) concentration.
- rT3 measurements are not required for the diagnosis of sick euthyroid syndrome.
- It can be argued that thyroid function should not be assessed in patients who are acutely ill or hospitalized unless thyroid dysfunction is in the differential diagnosis of their presenting complaints (e.g., coma, heart failure) and other causes of their presenting complaint have already been excluded.
- Although it remains controversial, there is no unequivocal evidence that treating sick euthyroid syndrome with Na-L-thyroxine improves clinical outcomes.

Thyroid cancer

- Nonmalignant but neoplastic thyroid follicles are termed "follicular adenomas."
  - In follicular adenomas, neither the capsule nor the blood vessels are invaded by the tumor, which is in contrast to follicular carcinoma (see discussion below).
- Thyroid cancer can originate from:
  - Follicular cells;
  - C cells;

- ○ Lymphocytes; or
- ○ Cancer may be metastatic to the thyroid gland.
- Lymphomas can originate in the thyroid gland and are increased in frequency in people with autoimmune thyroid disease.
- Only rarely does metastatic cancer to the thyroid gland cause hypothyroidism.
- Thyroid cancers of follicular or C-cell origin are listed in Table 3.8.

Histology

- Papillary thyroid carcinoma (PTC) is the most common form of thyroid carcinoma of follicular cell origin.
  - ○ The histologic diagnosis of PTC is dependent on the recognition of

Table 3.8 Thyroid cancers.

Type	Description	Thyroid cancers, %	Circulating tumor marker
Follicular	Papillary thyroid carcinoma	75–85	Tg
	Follicular carcinoma	10–20	Tg
	Anaplastic	<5	None
C cell	Medullary thyroid carcinoma	~5	Calcitonin

Tg, thyroglobulin.

folded nuclei, pseudoinclusions, and psammoma bodies.
- Follicular carcinoma is differentiated from follicular adenoma by the invasion of the capsule or blood vessels by carcinomas.
- Anaplastic thyroid carcinoma has a very poor prognosis.
  - ○ Most often occurs in the elderly population
  - ○ Usually has an average survival of only ~6 months following diagnosis
  - ○ Anaplasia in anaplastic thyroid carcinoma is histologically manifested as:
    - Spindled cells;
    - Giant cells;
    - Pleomorphism;
    - Mitoses; and
    - Necrosis.
- Medullary thyroid carcinoma (MTC) is characterized by amyloid deposits within the tumor.
  - ○ The amyloid deposition is procalcitonin.

- There are Hürthle cell variants of the thyroid follicular adenomas or carcinomas.
  - Hürthle cells are also described as oxyphilic or oncocytic cells.
  - Brightly eosinophilic (pink) and granular cytoplasm results from an extraordinarily large number of mitochondria.
  - The function of Hürthle cells is unknown.

Differentiated thyroid carcinomas

- PTC and follicular carcinoma can be described as differentiated thyroid carcinomas (DTCs).
- DTC has a relatively good prognosis.
  - Therapy is beyond the scope of this guide.
- Both of these cancers can secrete Tg.
- If surgical thyroidectomy is complete, then Tg levels should become undetectable.
  - However, if Tg Ab are present then the Tg value is unreliable unless measured by RIA or mass spectrometry.
- If there is residual thyroid tissue or DTC tumor remaining after surgery, then Tg can be detectable and the cancer may require continued therapy (e.g., radioactive iodine).
- Following surgery for a DTC, Na-L-thyroxine is prescribed to suppress the TSH level because TSH may be trophic for DTC.
- Because suppressed TSH may lead to a suppressed Tg level, the thyroid gland should be stimulated postoperatively prior to measuring the Tg level.
  - Stimulation is achieved by the use of recombinant TSH (thyrotropin alpha, which is very expensive) or, more commonly, Na-L-thyroxine withdrawal prior to testing (which can cause hypothyroid symptoms).

Medullary thyroid carcinoma

- Medullary thyroid carcinomas (MTCs) arise from thyroid parafollicular cells (also referred to as "C-cells") and secrete calcitonin.
  - MTC can be sporadic (80% of cases) or familial (20% of cases).
  - Familial MTC can occur as isolated MTC or as part of type 2 multiple endocrine neoplasia (MEN).
    - 100% of patients with type 2 MEN will develop MTC, whereas 50% will develop pheochromocytoma.
    - MEN type 2: Results from mutations in the *RET* proto-oncogene. The age at which MTC could occur can be estimated from the

specific RET codon affected and can direct the urgency for thyroidectomy.

- MEN types 2A and B: Distinguished by the presence of mucosal neuromas and a marfanoid habitus in type 2B.

Newborn screening for thyroid dysfunction

- Newborn screening for the detection of congenital hypothyroidism is universally accepted and recommended.
- Screening children outside of the newborn period who are asymptomatic for thyroid dysfunction is controversial.
  - Children with Trisomy 21 have an increased risk of autoimmune disease. HT occurs in up to 40% of children with Down syndrome and American Academy of Pediatrics recommends at least a TSH level be obtained at 6 and 12 months of life then annually.
- The U.S. Preventive Services Task Force on the matter states:
  - "The evidence is insufficient to recommend for or against routine screening for thyroid disease in adults."

Conclusion

- Although thyroid disease usually presents as dysfunction and/or goiter or nodules, the spectrum of thyroid disease is often bewildering because thyroid hormone affects many processes and thyroid dysfunction has many causes and intricacies.
- Untreated thyroid disease can produce significant symptoms and can be life-threatening in certain circumstances.
- Because of the generally good prognosis of DTC with proper therapy, there are an increasing number of people in the general population who will have a history of DTC.
- The laboratory plays a major role in the diagnosis, therapy and monitoring of thyroid disease.

Suggested reading

Francis GL, Waguespack SG, Bauer AJ, Angelos P, Benvenga S, Cerutti JM, Dinauer CA, Hamilton J, Hay ID, Luster M, Parisi MT, Rachmiel M, Thompson GB, Yamashita S, American Thyroid Association Guidelines Task Force. Management guidelines for children with thyroid nodules and differentiated thyroid cancer. Thyroid 2015;25(7):716–59. https://doi.org/10.1089/thy.2014.0460. PMID: 25900731. PMCID: PMC4854274.

Haugen BR. Drugs that suppress TSH or cause central hypothyroidism. Best Pract Res Clin Endocrinol Metab 2009;23(6):793–800. https://doi.org/10.1016/j.beem.2009.08.003. PMID: 19942154. PMCID: PMC2784889.

Lazarus JH, Bestwick JP, Channon S, Paradice R, Maina A, Rees R, et al. Antenatal thyroid screening and childhood cognitive function. N Engl J Med 2012;366:493–501.

Metwalley KA, Farghaly HS. Graves' disease in children: an update. Clin Med Insights Endocrinol Diabetes 2023;3(16), 11795514221150615. https://doi.org/10.1177/11795514221150615. PMID: 37151843. PMCID: PMC10161304.

U.S. Preventive Services Task Force. Thyroid dysfunction: screening., 2015, https://www.uspreventiveservicestaskforce.org/uspstf/recommendation/thyroid-dysfunction-screening.

U.S. Preventive Services Task Force. Thyroid cancer: screening., 2017, https://www.uspreventiveservicestaskforce.org/uspstf/recommendation/thyroid-cancer-screening.

Winter WE, Schatz D, Bertholf RL. The thyroid: Pathophysiology and thyroid function testing. In: Burtis C, Ashwood E, Bruns D, editors. Tietz textbook of clinical chemistry and molecular diagnostics. 5th ed. St. Louis, MO: Elsevier Saunders; 2012. p. 1905–44.

CHAPTER 4

Adrenal gland

Physiology

Adrenal cortex and medulla

- The adrenal gland is composed of a (Fig. 4.1):
  - Cortex and
  - Medulla.
- The cortex contains three layers:
  - Glomerulosa;
  - Fasciculata; and
  - Reticularis.
- The hormonal product of the glomerulosa is aldosterone (Fig. 4.2), the major mineralocorticoid in humans.
- The hormonal products of the fasciculata and the reticularis (Fig. 4.2) are cortisol, the major glucocorticoid in humans, and the adrenal androgens, dehydroepiandrosterone (DHEA) and androstenedione, respectively.
  - The major hormonal product of the medulla is epinephrine.

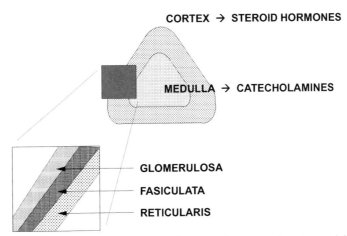

Fig. 4.1 The adrenal gland is composed of a cortex (outer layer) and a medulla (inner layer). The cortex is further composed of three layers: glomerulosa (the source of the mineralocorticoid aldosterone), the fasciculata, and reticularis (the sources of glucocorticoid cortisol and the adrenal androgens dehydroepiandrosterone and androstenedione). The catecholamine epinephrine is the major product of the medulla.

Quick Guide to Endocrinology
https://doi.org/10.1016/B978-0-443-14135-5.00004-1

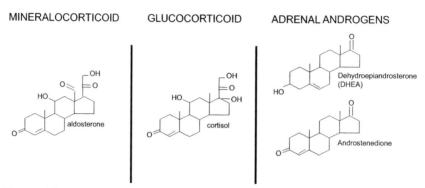

Fig. 4.2 These are the chemical formulas for the mineralocorticoid aldosterone, the glucocorticoid cortisol, and the adrenal androgens DHEA and androstenedione. DHEA, dehydroepiandrosterone.

Adrenal cortical hormones

- Mineralocorticoids act on the distal convoluted tubules (DCTs) and collecting ducts of the nephron.
  - They reabsorb sodium in exchange for potassium and hydrogen ions (Fig. 4.3).
    - As sodium is reabsorbed, so is water, maintaining blood pressure and vascular tone.
- Glucocorticoids are stress hormones (e.g., a hormone that is secreted at the time of psychological or physiological stress). Glucocorticoids:
  - Act to raise blood glucose (by increasing gluconeogenesis and causing insulin resistance);
  - Maintain blood pressure and cardiac output;
  - Stabilize lysosomal membranes; and
  - Are catabolic.
  - In supraphysiological doses, administered glucocorticoids are immunosuppressive and produce a variety of adverse side effects (see Cushing syndrome below).
- Adrenal androgens stimulate development of axillary and pubic hair (see Chapter 5 for a further discussion of adrenal androgens) (Fig. 4.4). In males, the effects of testosterone on stimulating axillary and pubic hair outweighs the effects of the adrenal androgens under normal circumstances.

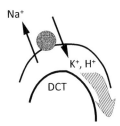

Fig. 4.3 The actions of mineralocorticoids on the DCT and collecting ducts (not shown) are to increase sodium (Na⁺) reabsorption, and waste potassium (K⁺) and hydrogen ions (H⁺). DCT, distal convoluted tube.

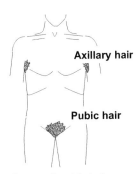

Fig. 4.4 The distribution of axillary and pubic hair.

Adrenal medulla

- Like cortisol, epinephrine is a stress hormone.
- As a catecholamine, epinephrine:
  - Raises blood glucose (by stimulating glycogenolysis, gluconeogenesis, and causing insulin resistance);
  - Increases heart rate and cardiac contractility;
  - Produces vasoconstriction elevating blood pressure;
  - Reduces urine output through its vasoconstrictor action on the arterial bed of the kidney; and
  - Causes sweating, increased alertness, and anxiety.

Steroid physiology and the regulation of secretion of the adrenocortical hormones

- Mineralocorticoids (i.e., aldosterone) are controlled by the renin-angiotensin system (Fig. 4.5).

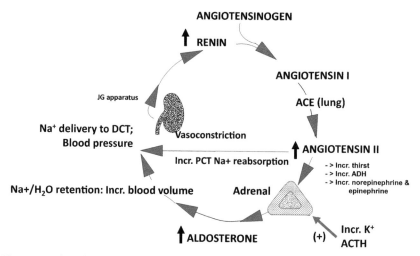

Fig. 4.5 With either a decline in the delivery of sodium (Na^+) to the DCT or reduced perfusion pressure of the afferent arteriole (both monitored by the Juxtaglomerular [JG] apparatus), renin is released. The enzymatic activity of renin converts angiotensinogen to angiotensin I. Angiotensin I is converted to angiotensin II via the action of ACE that is expressed in the lung. Angiotensin II is a powerful vasoconstrictor, as well as, increasing the PCT reabsorption of Na^+, increasing thirst, increasing ADH release, increasing norepinephrine and epinephrine levels and, very importantly, increasing aldosterone secretion from the adrenal cortex. Aldosterone increases Na^+ and water reabsorption to increase circulating volume, thus increasing systemic perfusion. This completes the negative feedback loop. ACE, angiotensin-converting enzyme; ACTH, adrenocorticotropic hormone; ADH, antidiuretic hormone; DCT, distal convoluted tube; incr., increased; JG, juxtaglomerular apparatus; PCT, proximal convoluted tubule.

- The pathway from cholesterol to aldosterone is as follows (enzymes in parentheses) (Fig. 4.6):
  - Cholesterol—(CYP11A) → pregnenolone
  - Pregnenolone—(3 beta-hydroxysteroid dehydrogenase and delta^4,5-isomerase) → progesterone
  - Progesterone—(21-hydroxylase   [CYP21]) → desoxycorticosterone (DOC)
  - DOC—(CYP11B2, an 11 beta-hydroxylase) → corticosterone
  - Corticosterone—(CYP11B2) → 18-hydroxycorticosterone
  - 18-Hydroxycorticosterone—(CYP11B2) → aldosterone
- Renin is released by the juxtaglomerular (JG) apparatus of the nephron when there is:

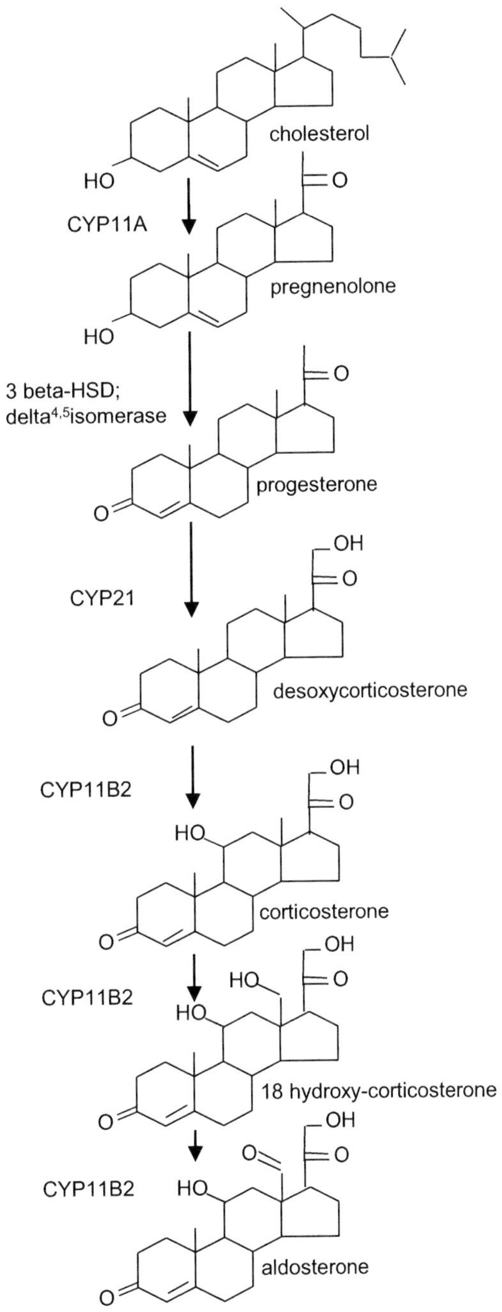

Fig. 4.6 The biochemical pathway for the synthesis of aldosterone. See text for details.

- ○ Decreased perfusion pressure of the glomerular afferent arterioles and/or
- ○ Decreased sodium concentration of the fluid in the DCT.
- As an enzyme, renin converts angiotensinogen to angiotensin I.
- Angiotensin I is converted to angiotensin II by the enzyme angiotensin-converting enzyme (ACE) present in the vasculature of the lung.
- Angiotensin II is a very powerful vasoconstrictor that also stimulates:
  - ○ Vasopressin release;
  - ○ Catecholamine release;
  - ○ Increased thirst; and
  - ○ Increased sodium reabsorption through the proximal convoluted tubule (PCT).
- Of great importance, angiotensin II regulates the release of aldosterone by the adrenal cortex.
- Whereas, cortisol is controlled by the hypothalamic-pituitary-adrenal axis (Fig. 4.7).

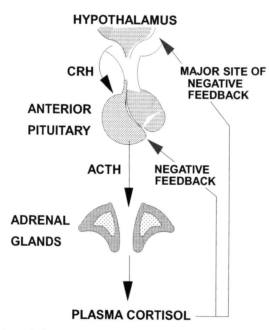

Fig. 4.7 The hypothalamus releases CRH that travels to the anterior pituitary corticotrophs via the hypothalamic-pituitary portal system. In response to CRH, the corticotrophs secrete ACTH (also known as corticotropin) that stimulates the secretion of cortisol from the adrenal cortex. The major site of negative feedback is at the hypothalamus. To a lesser degree, cortisol feeds back negatively at the level of the pituitary. ACTH, adrenocorticotropic hormone; CRH, corticotropin-releasing hormone.

- The hypothalamus releases corticotropin–releasing hormone (CRH), which is under control of the central nervous system (CNS).
- CRH reaches the anterior pituitary via the hypothalamic–pituitary portal system.
- By binding to CRH receptors on corticotrophs of the anterior pituitary, the corticotrophs secrete adrenocorticotropic hormone (ACTH, also known as corticotropin).
- ACTH is the proteolytic cleavage product of the large precursor molecule pro-opiomelanocortin (POMC) (Fig. 4.8).

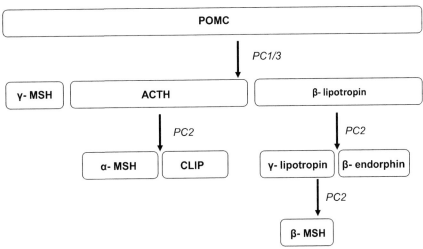

Fig. 4.8 Processing of POMC into ACTH and other downstream products is carried out by pro-hormone convertase enzymes. POMC, pro-opiomelanocortin; ACTH, adrenocorticotropic hormone; PC1/3, pro-hormone convertase 1/3; PC2, pro-hormone convertase 2; MSH, melanocyte stimulating hormone; CLIP, corticotropin-like intermediate peptide.

- ACTH stimulates the production and release of cortisol.
- Similar to other steroid hormones, cortisol:
  - Is produced as needed;
  - Diffuses out of the cell;
  - Circulates systemically (partially bound to a binding protein); and
  - Binds to cell surface and intracellular receptors.
- Steroid hormones are not stored in endocrine cells.
  - In contrast to protein hormones, thyroid hormone, and catecholamines that are synthesized and stored for secretion

- The pathway from cholesterol to cortisol is as follows (enzymes in parentheses) (Fig. 4.9):
    - Cholesterol—(CYP11A) → pregnenolone
    - Pregnenolone—(3 beta-hydroxysteroid dehydrogenase and delta^{4,5}-isomerase) → progesterone—(CYP17) → 17-hydroxyprogesterone (17-OHP) (or)
    - Pregnenolone—(CYP17, a 17 alpha-hydroxylase) → 17-hydroxypregnenolone—(3 beta-hydroxysteroid dehydrogenase and delta^{4,5}-isomerase) → 17-OHP
    - 17-OHP—(CYP21) → 11-desoxycortisol
    - 11-Desoxycortisol—(CYP11B1, an 11 beta-hydroxylase) → cortisol

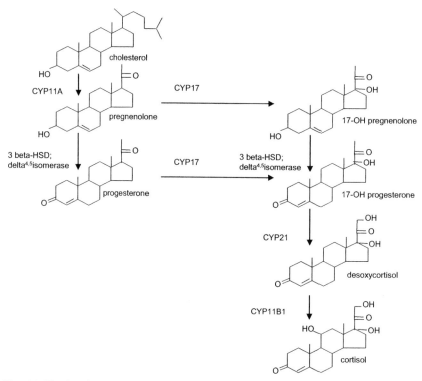

Fig. 4.9 The biochemical pathway for the synthesis of cortisol is depicted. See text for details.

- ACTH levels peak in the morning between 6 and 8 am, producing peak cortisol concentrations between 6 and 8 am. Therefore, ACTH and cortisol display diurnal variation, with the lowest levels at ~12 am (Fig. 4.10).

Many other hormones also have peak and trough times where knowing this is vital to assay timing. Similarly, disease states (e.g., Cushing syndrome) may skew diurnal variation.

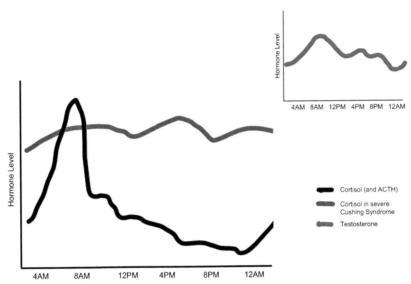

Fig. 4.10 Figure demonstrates variation in cortisol levels throughout a 24-h period in health (*black line*) and cushing syndrome (*red line*; where the diurinal variation is lost). In the upper right panel an additional hormone diurinal variation example is presented (for testosterone).

- 80–90% of cortisol is transported in the circulation by cortisol-binding globulin (CBG; also known as transcortin).
- The unbound (free) fraction of total cortisol is 2–3%, with ~7% loosely bound to albumin.
- The regulation of adrenal androgen production is not well understood.
- Production of the adrenal androgens is as follows (Fig. 4.11):
  o 17-hydroxypregnenolone—(CYP17, a 17,20-lyase) → DHEA
  o 17-hydroxyprogesterone—(CYP17, a 17,20-lyase) → androstenedione
  o DHEA—(3 beta-hydroxysteroid dehydrogenase and delta^{4,5}-isomerase) → androstenedione
- The entire adrenal cortex hormone synthesis pathway is depicted in Fig. 4.12 with the addition of the inactive metabolite of cortisol (cortisone), the sulfated (storage) form of DHEA (DHEAS), and estradiol and testosterone adrenal synthesis steps.

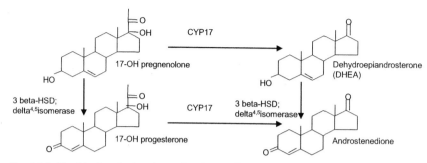

Fig. 4.11 The biochemical pathway for the synthesis of adrenal androgens is depicted. See text for details.

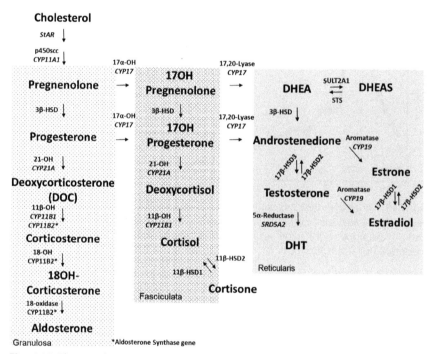

Fig. 4.12 The initial step in steroid hormone synthesis in the adrenal cortex is the conversion of cholesterol to pregnenolone (via StAR, p450scc, and CYP11A1 enzymes). The synthesis of aldosterone takes place in the glomerulosa. The synthesis of cortisol predominantly occurs in the fasciculata and the synthesis of adrenal androgens predominantly occurs in the reticularis. Cortisol acts on numerous organs and cells throughout the body. In the kidney, however, cortisol is converted to inactive cortisone via 11β-HSD2 to allow kidney-specific effects of aldosterone to be exerted. In the reticularis, adrenal androgens are converted to sex steroids (testosterone, DHT, estrone, and estradiol), though to a less extent than in the gonads. StAR, steroidogenic acute regulatory protein; p450scc, cholesterol side chain cleavage enzyme (also termed cholesterol desmolase); 3β-HSD, 3 beta-hydroxysteroid dehydrogenase; 21-OH, 21-hydroxylase; 11β-OH, 11β-hydroxylase; 18-OH, 18-hydroxylase; 17α-OH, 17α-hydroxylase; 11β-HSD1 (or 2), 11β-hydroxysteroid dehydrogenase 1 (or 2); SULT2A1, sulfotransferase (hydroxysteroid sulfotransferase 2A1); STS, steroid sulfatase; 17β-HSD, 17β-hydroxysteroid dehydrogenase.

Physiology and regulation of the secretion of the adrenomedullary catecholamines

- Epinephrine release by the adrenal medulla is controlled by the sympathetic nervous system.
- At times of stress, epinephrine is secreted.
- The precursor of catecholamines (as well as thyroid hormone and melanin) is phenylalanine (Fig. 4.13).

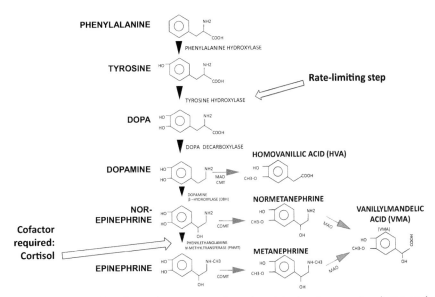

Fig. 4.13 Depicted is the pathway converting phenylalanine to norepinephrine and epinephrine (both of which can be measured in plasma or urine). Dopamine can be assayed in plasma or urine. HVA is a degradation product of dopamine that can be assayed in urine. Normetanephrine is a metabolite of norepinephrine and metanephrine is a metabolite of epinephrine. Collectively, these metabolites are known as the "metanephrines," which can be measured in plasma or urine. VMA is the common urinary metabolite of normetanephrine and metanephrine. DOPA, dihydroxyphenylalanine; HVA, homovanillic acid; VMA, vanillylmandelic acid.

- Phenylalanine hydroxylase converts phenylalanine to tyrosine.
- Tyrosine hydroxylase converts tyrosine of dihydroxyphenylalanine (DOPA).
- The action of DOPA decarboxylase on DOPA forms dopamine.
- Dopamine beta-hydroxylase converts dopamine to norepinephrine.
- Phenylethanolamine *N*-methyltransferase converts norepinephrine to epinephrine.

- In the urine, catecholamine metabolites can be detected and quantitated.
- Homovanillic acid (HVA) is the metabolite of dopamine (via the actions of monoamine oxidase [MAO] and catechol-amine-O-methyltransferase [COMT]).
- Normetanephrine is the immediate metabolite of norepinephrine (via the action of COMT).
- Metanephrine is the immediate metabolite of epinephrine (also via COMT).
- Normetanephrine and metanephrine can collectively be referred to as "metanephrines."
- Metanephrines are more stably secreted than epinephrine and norepinephrine.
- Normetanephrine and metanephrine are then metabolized to vanillyl-mandelic acid (VMA) via MAO.

Measurements

Adrenal cortex and related hormones

- ACTH is labile and specific pre-analytic considerations apply (e.g., blood is drawn into an ethylenediaminetetraacetic acid [EDTA] tube that is plastic or siliconized glass and the plasma is separated from the cells and frozen within 2 h of collection).
- Cortisol can be measured in:
  - Plasma;
  - Serum;
  - Urine; or
  - Saliva.
- Like ACTH, cortisol is most commonly measured by immunoassay.
  - A major concern regarding cortisol immunoassays is the specificity of the assay as, to varying degrees, other steroids can cross-react with cortisol.
  - Immunoassay specificity can be improved by extracting serum or urine prior to immunoassay. Some experts would argue that preparative extraction is an absolute requirement for urinary free cortisol (UFC) measurements.
  - Newer cortisol immunoassays have less cross reactivity and can detect cortisol at lower levels.
- Rarely, dexamethasone is measured to confirm compliance (during a dexamethasone suppression test) and exclude hypermetabolism in

compliant patients when they fail to demonstrate expected cortisol suppression during an overnight dexamethasone suppression test (see below).

- In cases of inborn errors in steroidogenesis, essentially any of the adrenal steroids can be measured at reference laboratories.
- Aldosterone can be measured in plasma or a timed urine sample.
- Renin is usually measured after the patient has been supine for ~20 min. Otherwise, the renin may be elevated because the subject has been upright.
  - Renin is measured as the plasma renin activity (PRA). Alternatively, the absolute renin concentration can be measured by immunoassay.
- Calculation of the plasma aldosterone to PRA ratio is informative in cases of hyperaldosteronism, separating primary from secondary states (see below).

Catecholamines

- Catecholamines can be measured in plasma or urine.
  - In urine, catecholamine excretion can be expressed per mg of creatinine; or
  - As an absolute amount excreted over the period of time of the collection (usually 24 h).
- Because of potential analytic inferences and the effects of stress and drugs on catecholamine secretion, proper pre-analytic preparation of the patient is important.
- Drugs that may interfere with accurate measurement of catecholamines should be discontinued prior to testing if safe, include:
  - Dopamine, norepinephrine, epinephrine,
  - Tricyclic antidepressants, SSRIs, SNRIs,
  - Non-selective alpha-blockers, beta-blockers,
  - MAOIs, sympathomimetics (including ephedrine, pseudoephedrine, amphetamines, albuterol)
  - Levodopa, calcium channel blockers, acetaminophen.
- For plasma measurements, patients must refrain from:
  - Eating, drinking caffeinated beverages;
  - Exercising, and
  - Using tobacco immediately prior to phlebotomy.
- Procedure for plasma measurements:
  - Insert an indwelling catheter to ensure that the patient is not stressed and keep the patient for 30 min prior to drawing the sample for catecholamine measurements.

- Patient should be supine and in a quiet environment for this time prior to drawing the sample from the indwelling catheter (after a blank sample is withdrawn to clear the line of diluent and anticoagulant).
  - Place the blood in a chilled EDTA-sodium metabisulfite tube.
  - Within 30 min of phlebotomy, the plasma is obtained using a refrigerated centrifuge and then immediately frozen.
- In plasma, dopamine, norepinephrine, epinephrine, and free metanephrines can be measured.
- In urine, dopamine, norepinephrine, epinephrine, and free metanephrines can be measured.

Deficiencies of adrenal steroids
Mineralocorticoid deficiency
- Aldosterone deficiency produces:
  - Hyponatremia;
  - Hyperkalemia, which can cause serious arrhythmias;
  - Acidosis; and
  - Hypovolemia, which can lead to hypotension and even shock.
- When combined with acute cortisol deficiency, acute aldosterone deficiency can cause an adrenal or Addisonian crisis that can be fatal (see below).
- Isolated aldosterone deficiency is rare and can result from inborn errors of metabolism, such as aldosterone synthase deficiency, or resistance to aldosterone can exist (pseudo-hypoaldosteronism).
- Aldosterone deficiency most commonly results from primary adrenal insufficiency (causes discussed below).
- The diagnosis is accomplished by finding low levels of plasma or urinary aldosterone and elevated renin concentrations, excluding the rare cases of renin deficiency (see below).
- Rarely, renin deficiency will cause aldosterone deficiency.
  - Renin deficiency can develop in people with long-standing diabetes mellitus.
- If cortisol deficiency has been diagnosed and the potassium is elevated, aldosterone measurements are usually not necessary because the clinical picture fits that of primary adrenal insufficiency (i.e., Addison disease).
- Aldosterone deficiency is treated with oral 9-alpha fluorohydrocortisone (fludrocortisone).

o In infants, salt may be added to the diet. Acute deficiency can be treated with bolus IV fluids with normal saline (NS) and then replacement IV fluids [e.g., D5NS].

- Sufficiency of mineralocorticoid replacement is evidenced in:
  o Normal blood pressure and pulse;
  o Normal electrolytes (no hyponatremia or hyperkalemia); and a
  o PRA or renin concentration within the reference interval.

Glucocorticoid deficiency

- Cortisol deficiency produces a variety of findings (Table 4.1).

Table 4.1 Characteristic findings resulting from glucocorticoid deficiency.

Malaise, tiredness, lassitude, weakness, and easy fatigability
Gastrointestinal upset (e.g., nausea, vomiting, diarrhea)
Weight loss
Hypovolemia and hyponatremia
Pallor (from anemia)
When severe deficiency is present: hypoglycemia, hypotension, and impaired cardiac output
Hyperpigmentation (*in cases of primary adrenal insufficiency from elevated ACTH levels*)

ACTH, adrenocorticotropic hormone.

- Deficiency of ACTH (due to disease or dysfunction of the hypothalamus, the hypothalamic-pituitary portal system or pituitary) leads to cortisol deficiency but aldosterone secretion is maintained.
- ACTH deficiency causes "secondary (or central) adrenal insufficiency."
- Diseases of the adrenal cortex usually impair both cortisol and aldosterone secretion.
- Deficiency of both hormones is termed Addison disease (also called primary adrenal insufficiency).
- Table 4.2 lists causes of primary adrenal insufficiency.
- There are two major autoimmune polyglandular syndromes (APSs) that include autoimmune primary adrenal insufficiency:
  o Type 1
    ▪ Also termed autoimmune polyendocrinopathy candidiasis ectodermal dystrophy (APECED)
    ▪ Occurrence of Addison disease or adrenal autoantibodies plus mucocutaneous candidiasis and/or hypo-parathyroidism
    ▪ Autosomal recessive disorder that results from mutations in the *AIRE* gene (AIRE = autoimmune regulator)

- Onset can be in infancy
- Equal frequency in boys and girls
  ○ Type 2
    - Occurrence of Addison disease or adrenal autoantibodies plus type 1 diabetes mellitus and/or autoimmune thyroid disease (HT or GD)
    - Polygenic inheritance associated with human leukocyte antigen (HLA) genotypes.
    - Type 3 APS is the same HLA risk and disease conditions except without Addison disease.
    - Disorder is polygenic and affects women more often than men.
    - Onset is in childhood or adulthood

Table 4.2 Causes of Addison disease (primary adrenal insufficiency).

Immune/autoimmune
Autoimmune (isolated Addison disease or associated with an autoimmune polyglandular syndrome)
Infectious (e.g., HIV infection, tuberculosis)
Inflammatory (e.g., sarcoidosis)
Vascular
Hemorrhagic (e.g., trauma)
Coagulopathic (e.g., Waterhouse-Friderichsen syndrome or sepsis)
Venous obstruction (e.g., adrenal venous thrombosis, heparin-induced thrombosis, antiphospholipid antibody syndrome)
Metabolic
Inborn errors of metabolism (e.g., 21-hydroxylase deficiency congenital adrenal hyperplasia [CAH], congenital adrenal hypoplasia, adrenoleukodystrophy)
Drugs
Blockers of steroid synthesis (e.g., mitotane, aminoglutethimide, trilostane, ketoconazole, metyrapone)
Glucocorticoid receptor blockers (e.g., mifepristone)
Anatomic/Infiltrative
Developmental disorders (e.g., congenital adrenal hypoplasia, aplasia)
Postadrenalectomy
Infiltrative (e.g., tumor, amyloid)

HIV, human immunodeficiency virus.

- Diagnostically, the best test of cortisol sufficiency is to measure cortisol at the time of adrenal crisis (i.e., severe illness) when the cortisol should be above 15 μg/dL.
  ○ Values <15 μg/dL (lower cutoffs may be appropriate depending on the assay) are consistent with cortisol deficiency.

- In the absence of adrenal crisis, cortisol can be measured 30 and 60 min (or 45 min for single sampling protocols) following the intravenous (IV) or intramuscular (IM) injection of cosyntropin at either high or low-dose depending on the suspected lesion (Fig. 4.14).

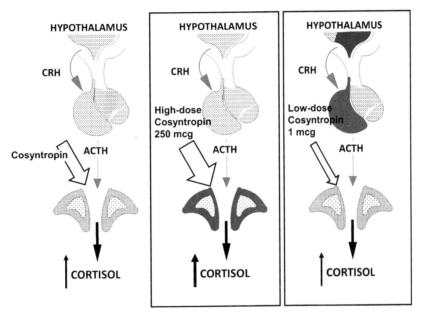

Fig. 4.14 In the cosyntropin stimulation test, cosyntropin is administered and the adrenal gland's cortisol response is measured. A deficient response is observed in cases of CRH deficiency, ACTH deficiency, or primary adrenal failure. Typically, a higher dose of Cosyntropin is administered in cases of primary adrenal insufficiency as a larger stimulus is needed to determine if a "damaged" adrenal gland can produce a cortisol response during times of stress. A smaller, but still supratherapeutic, dose of cosyntropin is often administered when suspicion of secondary (or central) adrenal insufficiency is high. This test is more sensitive but less specific for adrenal insufficiency (i.e., more false positives may occur). Without continuous stimulation of the adrenal cortex by endogenous ACTH, the adrenal glands can atrophy over time. ACTH, adrenocorticotropic hormone; CRH, corticotropin-releasing hormone.

- Cosyntropin is the synthetic polypeptide that includes the first 24 amino acids of ACTH.
- Peak cortisol should normally reach ≥ 15 μg/dL following cosyntropin.
  - Values <15 μg/dL may be consistent with cortisol deficiency.
  - The change in cortisol is normally >7–10 μg/dL, but the absolute cortisol is the better measure of cortisol deficiency.

- Although a low morning cortisol (e.g., <2–3 µg/dL) is consistent with cortisol deficiency, this is a later finding in the natural history of Addison disease than the failure of cortisol to respond to cosyntropin.
  - However, if the morning cortisol is >15 µg/dL and the index of suspicion for Addison disease is low, Addison disease is unlikely.
  - Nevertheless, if adrenal autoantibodies are present or if there is an autoimmune polyglandular syndrome, future surveillance (e.g., repeat cosyntropin testing) is indicated.
- Cortisol can also be stimulated by the induction of hypoglycemia via the IV injection of insulin. This test is labor intensive and not often performed.
  - This is an invasive and potentially dangerous test.
  - Stable IV access (for the administration of glucose and glucagon) is necessary.
- If mineralocorticoid and glucocorticoid deficiency both exist, there is no question that there is primary adrenal insufficiency.
  - However, if mineralocorticoid secretion is intact (with a normal renin level), the tests above do not distinguish primary adrenal insufficiency from secondary adrenal insufficiency (ACTH deficiency).
    - ACTH level that is elevated due to lack of negative feedback from cortisol can distinguish these forms.
  - In the very early stages of mineralocorticoid deficiency, increases in PRA/renin concentration are the first laboratory abnormalities.
- In cases of primary adrenal insufficiency, the ACTH is generally elevated.
  - However, because of the wide diurnal variation in ACTH (and cortisol), isolated ACTH measurements may be difficult to interpret.
    - In other words, a seemingly elevated ACTH does not confirm the diagnosis of primary adrenal insufficiently and the measurement of cortisol during a crisis or after stimulation via cosyntropin or hypoglycemia is still required.
- Serologic markers of autoimmune adrenalitis include adrenal cytoplasmic autoantibodies (ACAs) measured by indirect immunofluorescence and 21-hydroxylase autoantibodies measured by immunoassay.
- Cortisol deficiency is treated with any of a variety of oral glucocorticoids, such as:
  - Hydrocortisone;
  - Prednisone; or
  - Dexamethasone.

- The most physiologic replacement is hydrocortisone especially during childhood growth (which is the pharmacologic name for cortisol).
    - Requires administration at least twice daily and possibly three times per day for the best outcome.
- Glucocorticoid overtreatment can produce Cushing syndrome.
- Sufficiency of glucocorticoid replacement is evidenced as:
    - Improvement in clinical symptomatology;
    - Normal blood pressure; and
    - Normal growth

Congenital adrenal hyperplasia

- Congenital adrenal hyperplasia (CAH) describes a family of inborn errors of metabolism where there is impaired cortisol synthesis. In turn, in response to elevated ACTH levels as a consequence of hypocortisolemia, there is hyperplasia of the adrenal cortex.
    - Inherited as an autosomal recessive trait, 21-hydroxylase enzyme deficiency (a loss-of-function mutation in CYP21, a P450 enzyme) causes 95% of cases of CAH.
        - 21-Hydroxylase deficiency impairs the conversion of 17-OHP to 11-deoxycortisol (recall that 11-deoxy-cortisol is the immediate precursor of cortisol; Fig. 4.15). Therefore, 17-OHP levels become elevated.

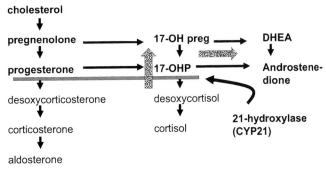

Fig. 4.15 In 21-hydroxylase deficiency CAH (the block is indicated by the gray horizontal bar), there is an accumulation of the cortisol precursors 17-OH preg and 17-OHP that are shunted to production of the adrenal androgens DHEA and androstenedione. The gray spotted arrow indicates the rising concentration of 17-OHP in untreated cases of 21-hydroxylase deficiency CAH. 17-OH, 17-hydroxypregnenolone; 17-OH preg, 17-hydroxypregnenolone; 17-OHP, and 17-hydroxyprogesterone; CAH, congenital adrenal hyperplasia; DHEA, dehydroepiandrosterone.

- Because of this inborn error with elevated ACTH stimulation of the cortex, as well as increased 17-OHP, adrenal androgen concentrations rise (specifically androstenedione).
- In its milder forms, aldosterone production in 21-hydroxylase deficiency CAH is not pathologically decreased; rather, only cortisol is decreased. In its more severe forms, aldosterone production in 21-hydroxylase deficiency CAH is decreased, thus causing potentially serious salt-wasting and even Addisonian crises.
- The second most common cause of CAH is 11 beta-hydroxylase deficiency, which is also inherited as an autosomal recessive trait (Fig. 4.16).
  ○ Increased androgens in utero cause a difference of sexual development (DSD) in females, similar to what is seen in 21-hydroxylase deficiency CAH.
  ○ However, no salt-wasting crisis occurs because of elevated levels of DOC (desoxycorticosterone), a salt-retaining hormone. Hypertension with hypokalemia can develop in infancy or childhood. In addition, boys may experience precocious puberty in either of these forms of CAH.

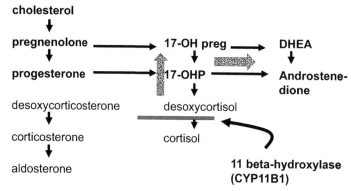

Fig. 4.16 In 11 beta-hydroxylase (CYP11B1) deficiency CAH (the block is indicated by the gray horizontal bar), there is an accumulation of the cortisol precursors including 17-OH preg and 17-OHP that are shunted to production of the adrenal androgens DHEA and androstenedione. The gray speckled arrow indicates the rising concentration of 17-OHP in untreated cases. 17-OH, 17-hydroxypregnenolone; 17-OH preg, 17-hydroxypregnenolone; 17-OHP, and 17-hydroxyprogesterone; CAH, congenital adrenal hyperplasia; DHEA, dehydroepiandrosterone.

21-Hydroxylase deficiency in females
- 21-Hydroxylase deficiency produces a DSD with ambiguous genitalia.
  ○ The consequence of the virilizing effects of increased adrenal androgen concentrations in utero

- Several clinical variations of 21-hydroxylase deficiency CAH exist, possibly influencing (Table 4.3):
  - Plasma electrolytes;
  - Genital development (producing a DSD);
  - The regularity of menstruation beginning with adolescence; and
  - Growth and adult height.

Table 4.3 Clinical varieties of 21-hydroxylase deficiency CAH in women.

Hyponatremia/ hyperkalemia[a]		Causes a DSD	Causes hyperandrogenism, impaired menstruation[a]
Simple-virilizing	No	Yes	Yes
Salt-wasting	Yes	Yes	Yes
Late-onset	No	No	Yes

[a]If untreated.
CAH, congenital adrenal hyperplasia; DSD, difference of sexual development (see Chapter 5).

- In the simple-virilizing variant, salt-wasting crisis (i.e., Addisonian crisis) does not occur because aldosterone levels are not pathologically decreased.
- Effects of this disorder are predominantly in utero virilization and ambiguous genitalia.
- Left untreated, androgens stimulate increased growth.
  - Premature fusion of the epiphyses may occur and ultimately cause short stature.
- In the salt-wasting variant, hyperkalemia, severe acidosis, hypovolemia, hypotension, and even Addisonian crisis can develop in addition to hyponatremia and hypoglycemia (these latter two findings are observed with cortisol deficiency).
  - Therefore, it can be fatal if not recognized and treated, whereas simple virilizing 21-hydroxylase CAH is not immediately fatal if left untreated.
- In the late-onset variant (also termed non-classical CAH), in utero hyperandrogenism and virilization does not occur because the degree of enzyme deficiency is mild.
  - However, hyperandrogenism does occur near the time of puberty and may cause hirsutism, absent or irregular menses, and even virilization.
- The diagnosis of 21-hydroxylase deficiency is based on:
  - Compatible clinical history;
  - Electrolyte abnormalities; and an
  - Elevated morning 17-OHP level.
  - Molecular testing can be considered for the *CYP21A2* gene or others in the pathway.

21-Hydroxylase deficiency in males

- 21-Hydroxylase deficiency in males does not produce a DSD.
  - Increased androgens in utero can cause some increase in the pigmentation of the male external genitalia.
- The male equivalent of "simple-virilizing 21-hydroxylase deficiency CAH" does not present in the immediate new-born period.
  - However, either in infancy or early childhood, excess adrenal androgens (e.g., androstenedione) cause precocious puberty with accelerated growth, increased penile size, and the development of axillary and pubic hair.
- Because the adrenal glands are the source of the androgen, in the initial years of the precocious puberty, the testes do not enlarge.
- Adult height can be reduced because of early epiphyseal fusion.
- Salt-wasting 21-hydroxylase deficiency CAH can be fatal in newborn males if not recognized and aggressively treated. It is also fatal if left untreated in female infants but it is more likely that the condition will be detected in females because of the recognition of a DSD immediately following birth.

Treatment of 21-hydroxylase deficiency

- Deficiencies of cortisol and aldosterone are treated as noted above.
- If an individual with apparent simple-virilizing CAH has an elevated PRA/renin concentration, mineralocorticoid replacement is advised.
- Achievement of androgen suppression is monitored by measuring androstenedione.
  - The sampling time is immaterial for androstenedione.
  - Successful glucocorticoid therapy suppresses androstenedione and symptoms of hyperandrogenism without producing glucocorticoid excess and Cushing syndrome.
  - If 17-OHP is measured, the sample should be obtained in the morning as 17-OHP displays diurnal variation. However, 17-OHP is not an ideal marker of therapeutic efficacy because normalization of the 17-OHP level has been shown to cause Cushingoid features indicating overtreatment with glucocorticoids.

Adrenal androgen deficiency

- There are no diseases of adrenal androgen deficiency.

Adrenal steroid excesses

Mineralocorticoid excess

- Aldosterone excess causes sodium and water retention that can cause volume expansion (short term) and hypertension.
- Excessive loss of potassium causes hypokalemia and excess loss of hydrogen ion causes a hypochloremic alkalosis.
- Hypokalemia can cause weakness and serious cardiac arrhythmias.
  - The most common presentation of pathologic hyperaldosteronism is hypokalemic, alkalotic hypertension.
- Hyperaldosteronism is also a diagnostic consideration when hypertension is resistant to routine therapy.
- The two most common causes of aldosterone excess are:
  - Aldosterone-producing adenoma (APA, also known as Conn syndrome) and
  - Bilateral adrenal hyperplasia (also known as idiopathic bilateral adrenal hyperplasia).
- APA and bilateral adrenal hyperplasia are distinguished:
  - Radiologically and
  - By gross and microscopic examination of the adrenal glands.
- If there is the question whether excess aldosterone is coming from a single adrenal gland or two adrenal glands, a radiologist can cannulate each adrenal vein with measurement of aldosterone, or better yet, the aldosterone to cortisol ratio in each sample as well as in the inferior vena cava (IVC).
- By itself, the presence of a CT or MRI-detected mass in the adrenal does not establish the diagnosis of an APA (or any other specific pathology) because innocent, non-hyperfunctional adrenal adenomas (so called "incidentalomas") are common, being identified in 3%–10% of the general population.
- In APA, the aldosterone (or aldosterone to cortisol ratio) will be higher by at least 50% on one side (the affected side) versus the other (unaffected) side.
- Renin is suppressed in cases of primary hyperaldosteronism.
- The diagnosis of primary hyperaldosteronism is aided by the findings of:
  - Hypertension;
  - Hypokalemia;
  - Alkalosis; and
  - Suppressed PRA/renin concentration.

- Another aid in diagnosing primary hyperaldosteronism is the calculation of the aldosterone to PRA ratio.
  - The aldosterone/PRA ratio in primary hyperaldosteronism is usually ≥ 25.
- Secondary hyperaldosteronism is a compensatory, physiologic response to decreased tissue perfusion.
  - It results from heart failure or chronic hypovolemia from hypoalbuminemia with reduced oncotic pressure.
  - Hypoalbuminemia can result from the nephrotic syndrome or liver failure.
- Although hypokalemia and alkalosis do occur in cases of primary and secondary hyperaldosteronism, hypertension does not occur in secondary hyperaldosteronism unless caused by renal artery stenosis or renal disease.
- Less common than either Conn syndrome or bilateral adrenal hyperplasia, other causes of hypermineralocorticoidism, hypertension, and hypokalemia are:
  - DOC-secreting tumors;
  - Glucocorticoid-remediable hyperaldosteronism; and
  - Apparent mineralocorticoid excess (AME).
- Glucocorticoid-remediable hyperaldosteronism (also known as dexamethasone-suppressible hypertension) is an inborn error where a gene promoter responsive to ACTH has crossed over to control the transcription of the *aldosterone synthase* gene.
  - In this way, aldosterone comes under the control of ACTH.
  - By suppressing ACTH with physiologic amounts of glucocorticoids (e.g., dexamethasone), aldosterone production is reduced (note: dexamethasone lacks mineralocorticoid effects).
  - This disease is an autosomal dominant disorder with onset in childhood or infancy.
- AME results from an acquired or congenital deficiency of type 2 11 beta-hydroxysteroid dehydrogenase.
- Type 2 11 beta-hydroxysteroid dehydrogenase (11HSDB2) normally converts cortisol to cortisone in mineralocorticoid-responsive tissues (Fig. 4.17).
  - Cortisone does not bind to the mineralocorticoid receptor and is the inactive form of cortisol.
  - In this way, with the conversion of cortisol to cortisone, 11HSDB2 normally "protects" the mineralocorticoid receptor from cortisol.

- o 11HSDB2 is present in the brain, kidney, placenta and other organs to protect them from excess cortisol exposure.
- o The normal concentration of cortisol in the plasma is approximately 1000-fold higher than aldosterone.

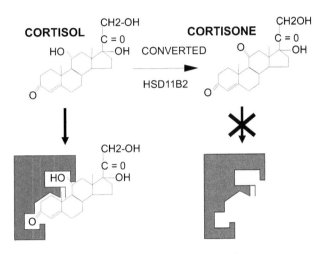

Fig. 4.17 Normally cortisol is converted to cortisone, which does not bind to the mineralocorticoid receptor. In apparent mineralocorticoid excess (AME), cortisol is not converted to cortisone and cortisol can then bind to the mineralocorticoid receptor causing a state of hypermineralocorticoidism.

- With a loss of 11HSDB2 activity, the mineralocorticoid receptor is not protected and cortisol binds to the mineralocorticoid receptor causing hypermineralocorticoidism.
- Elevated cortisol levels (as observed in Cushing syndrome) can produce a state of hypermineralocorticoidism when high cortisol levels overwhelm the "protective" action of 11HSDB2 in converting cortisol to cortisone.

Glucocorticoid excess

- Cortisol (or other glucocorticoid) excess produces Cushing syndrome (Table 4.4).
  - o Cushing syndrome is the term used to describe states of glucocorticoid excess.
  - o Cushing syndrome is most often exogenous from taking excess glucocorticoids.

Table 4.4 Characteristic features of Cushing syndrome.

Catabolism (including myopathy, stria, and osteoporosis with fractures)
Centripetal obesity with moon facies, thin arms and legs, and a dorsocervical fat pad
Hyperglycemia (from insulin resistance and increased gluconeogenesis)
Hirsutism in women (from glucocorticoid binding to the androgen receptor)
Hypertension, hypokalemia and alkalosis (from glucocorticoid binding to the mineralocorticoid receptor)
Immunosuppression with possible opportunistic infections
Psychiatric changes (e.g., emotional lability, depression, psychosis)

- Because of their powerful anti-inflammatory effects, glucocorticoids are often used to treat serious autoimmune and inflammatory disorders such as juvenile idiopathic arthritis and systemic lupus erythematosus.
  - High-dose glucocorticoids can also be used to treat some forms of cancer and are useful as powerful immunosuppressive agents in the setting of bone marrow or solid organ transplantation.
- Endogenous causes of Cushing syndrome include:
  - Anterior pituitary adenomas secreting ACTH (corticotropinomas causing "Cushing disease");
  - Adrenal tumors producing cortisol; and the
  - Rare ectopic production of ACTH (or less commonly CRH) from a tumor, driving hypercortisolism (i.e., ectopic ACTH, ectopic CRH).
- Adrenal tumors causing hypercortisolism include:
  - Glucocorticoid-producing adenomas (most common);
  - Glucocorticoid-producing carcinomas;
  - Bilateral micronodular hyperplasia; and
  - Bilateral macronodular hyperplasia.
  - These disorders are distinguished radiologically and by gross and microscopic examination of the adrenal glands.
  - If there is the question of whether excess cortisol is coming from a single adrenal gland or both adrenal glands, a radiologist can cannulate each adrenal vein and measure cortisol in each adrenal as well as the IVC (see the previous discussion of APA versus bilaterial adrenal hyperplasia). In small children, however, this procedure can be challenging due to the small adrenal vein size.
- The three stages to establishing the diagnosis of endogenous Cushing syndrome (see below) are:
  - (1) Exogenous Cushing syndrome must be excluded by history and review (if necessary) of pharmacy records;

- o (2) Biochemical confirmation (or denial) of cortisol excess; and
- o (3) Identification of the reason for the excess production of cortisol (e.g., corticotropinoma [Cushing disease] versus ectopic ACTH/CRH versus adrenal tumor).
- There are still other approaches to the diagnosis of Cushing syndrome; however, the approaches presented here are generally reliable and extensively utilized by clinicians.
- *Stage 1*
  - o Requires that the physician caring for the patient excludes an exogenous source of excess glucocorticoid before a formal biochemical work-up is pursued for endogenous Cushing syndrome.
  - o Glucocorticoids can be taken orally, or they can be absorbed topically from the lung or the skin, or injected into joints (the latter being less common).
  - o Cutaneous absorption of glucocorticoids is accelerated in skin conditions where the integrity of the skin has been reduced (e.g., severe atopic dermatitis).
- *Stage 2*
  - o Biochemical confirmation of excess cortisol involves any one or combination of the following three tests:
    - 24-h urinary free cortisol (UFC);
    - Overnight dexamethasone suppression test; and
    - Midnight cortisol (usually salivary).
  - o In patients with true endogenous Cushing syndrome, UFC is two to three times the upper limit of the reference interval.
  - o UFC can be adjusted for body mass index, which could be especially helpful in the evaluation of pediatric patients.
  - o In the overnight dexamethasone suppression test, 1 mg of dexamethasone (0.3 mg/m^2 in children) is taken orally at 10 pm to 12 am.
    - Cortisol is then measured at 8 am the next morning.
  - o Normally, morning cortisol is suppressed (i.e., $<1.8 \text{ μg/dL}$) after pm dexamethasone (dexamethasone is used in this test because it does not cross-react in the cortisol immunoassay).
  - o Cortisol is lowest usually at midnight when the plasma cortisol should be $<1.8 \text{ μg/dL}$. Higher values are abnormal.
  - o Because of the difficulty in performing a venipuncture on a sleeping patient, methods have been adapted to measure salivary cortisol. In such a case, the patient goes to sleep and sets an alarm for midnight. Once the patient awakes, they use a special kit to obtain saliva.

- ○ Often repeat samples are done on consecutive nights.
- ○ The properly obtained saliva sample is brought to the laboratory in the morning for analysis or sent out to a reference laboratory.
- ○ If the initial test (which can be any of the three tests) is normal (ruling against hypercortisolism) and the index of suspicion for Cushing syndrome is low, then Cushing syndrome has been excluded.
  - ▪ If the Index of suspicion for Cushing syndrome is high, any one of the three screening tests should be repeated as none of these tests has 100% accuracy.
- ○ If the initial test (which can be any one of the three tests) is abnormal (ruling for hypercortisolism):
  - ▪ Before proceeding to the invasive and expensive search for the cause of Cushing syndrome (stage 3), it is reasonable to confirm this with any one of the three tests that screen for hypercortisolism.
- • *Stage 3*
  - ○ There are two approaches to identifying the cause of the hypercortisolism:
    - ▪ A morning ACTH level that is elevated has a high sensitivity for ACTH-dependent Cushing disease.
    - ▪ High-dose dexamethasone suppression test is conducted to differentiate Cushing disease from ectopic ACTH secretion (which is rare in children).
      - ▪ High-dose dexamethasone suppression test: 120 µg/kg of dexamethasone (max 8 mg) is taken orally at 10 pm to 12 am. 2-Day administration protocols have also been used.
      - ▪ Cortisol is then measured at 8 am the next morning.
    - ▪ Causes of an abnormal screening test (stage 2) but suppression on low-dose dexamethasone are listed in Table 4.5.

Table 4.5 Causes of pseudo-Cushing syndrome.

Obesity
Depression
Stress
Alcoholism
Failure to take dexamethasone
Accelerated metabolism of dexamethasone during the overnight dexamethasone suppression test
Excess duration of urine collection (for urinary free cortisol measurement)
Contamination of saliva with blood (for salivary cortisol measurement)

- Such cases are sometimes referred to as pseudo-Cushing syndrome.
  - If there is no suppression on high-dose dexamethasone suppression test, the patient may have ectopic ACTH or CRH, or Cushing disease as 40% of people with Cushing disease do not suppress on high-dose dexamethasone.
  - If the plasma ACTH is suppressed: adrenal cortisol-secreting tumor is present.
  - If ACTH is not suppressed: ectopic ACTH or CRH is present.
  - If a cortisol-secreted adrenal tumor is suspected: Cannulation of the adrenal veins and cortisol measurements could confirm the presence of a cortisol-secreted adrenal tumor (i.e., the ratio of cortisol concentrations comparing one-side-to-other is 1.5) and the location (i.e., one side versus the other side adrenal).
  - In adults, adrenal adenomas are more common than adrenal carcinomas. While adrenal adenomas are also the most common adrenal tumor in children, adrenal carcinomas are most common in children under the age of 6 years.
  - If UFC suppression is not achieved, imaging such as inferior petrosal venous sinus sampling (IPSS) testing can be considered.
  - Inferior Petrosal Venous Sinus Sampling (IPSS)
    - The inferior petrosal sinuses receive venous drainage from the pituitary.
    - Both the left and right inferior petrosal sinuses are cannulated during this test along with the IVC (Fig. 4.18).

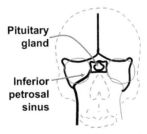

Fig. 4.18 This image depicts an anterior view of the cranium with the venous drainage of the pituitary passing into the inferior petrosal sinuses.

- Baseline ACTH levels at -30 and 0 min are drawn from all three sites.

- Ovine CRH is administered IV with samples drawn from all three sites at +2, +5, +10, and +30 min. Due to shortages of CRH, desmopressin was found to also be an effective stimulus during IPSS.
- If the ACTH is higher at baseline in either petrosal sinus and the ACTHs in the petrosal sinuses rise proportionately to a greater extent than the increase in IVC ACTH values, Cushing disease is confirmed.
- IPSS testing is not reliable in identifying if the corticotropinoma is on one side of the pituitary versus the other because venous drainage from the pituitary may be asymmetric.
- If the ACTH values at all sites are suppressed despite CRH administration, a cortisol-secreting adrenal tumor is likely present.
- If ACTH is measurable but does not respond to CRH and there is no gradient between the petrosal sinuses and the IVC, ectopic ACTH, or CRH is present.
- The diagnosis of Cushing syndrome is complex and difficult.
  - E.g., in rare cases, cortisol may only be secreted to excess during meals if the cortisol-secreting tumor expresses a receptor for incretins.
    - This is termed "gustatory" Cushing syndrome.
      Note: An overview of the diagnosis of Cushing syndrome is presented in Fig. 4.19.

Adrenal androgen excess
- This will be discussed in detail in Chapter 5; CAH is discussed above.
- Depending on the specific type of CAH a patient has, various steroids may be deficient (e.g., cortisol), but other steroids may be in great excess (e.g., 17-OHP, androstenedione).

Newborn screening for adrenal dysfunction

- Newborn screening for the detection of CAH allows for the early diagnosis of severe salt-wasting crises which can be fatal, and, of which boys are particular susceptible as there are no physical abnormalities (like ambiguous genitalia that baby girls often have) to promote further testing.
- Another disease leading to eventual adrenal insufficiency, which requires early treatment and monitoring to stave off death and improve neurologic outcomes, is adrenoleukodystrophy (ALD).

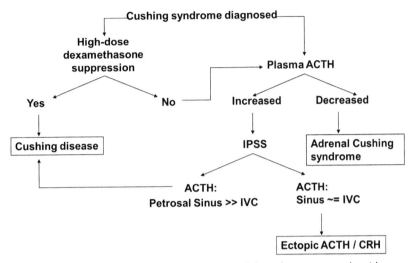

Fig. 4.19 Once Cushing syndrome is diagnosed based on repeated evidence of hypercortisolism (e.g., elevated 24-h UFC, failure of the 8 am cortisol to suppress to <1.8 µg/dL after 1 mg of dexamethasone at 10 pm to 12 am or elevated midnight salivary cortisol level), clinicians can elect to pursue further dexamethasone suppression testing or IPSS (inferior petrosal venous sinus sampling) testing. If there is cortisol suppression on high-dose dexamethasone administration, the diagnosis of Cushing disease is established. If there is no suppression, IPSS testing is pursued. IPSS testing begins by measuring the patient's ACTH on more than one occasion. If the ACTH is persistently suppressed, the diagnosis of adrenal Cushing syndrome is established. If the ACTH is persistently elevated, formal IPSS testing is pursued. If either of the inferior petrosal venous sinus ACTH levels are significantly elevated above IVC levels, Cushing disease is diagnosed. The differences in inferior petrosal venous sinus and IVC ACTH levels can be enhanced when ACTH is measured at all three sites after CRH administration. If the inferior petrosal venous sinus and IVC ACTH levels are equivalent, ectopic ACTH or CRH is diagnosed. UFC, urinary free cortisol; IPSS, inferior petrosal sinus sampling; ACTH, adrenocorticotropic hormone; IVC, inferior vena cava; CRH, corticotropin-releasing hormone.

- ○ ALD is an X-linked recessive disease that manifests in boys caused by variants in the *ABCD1* gene (ATP Binding Cassette Subfamily D Member 1).
- ○ Myelin abnormalities (due to a toxic buildup of very long chain fatty acids [VLCFA]) that progressively develop lead to impaired nerve signaling throughout the body. The adrenal cortex and the central nervous system are targeted.
- ○ Early monitoring for adrenal insufficiency and neurologic changes with the potential for bone marrow transplant before irreversible neurologic deterioration is an emerging therapy.

- Testing on newborn screen blood spot includes VLCFA levels. Reflex testing for the *ABDC1* gene mutation may also be done.
  - A majority of states in the United States have adopted this test but not all.

Adrenomedullary diseases

Excess secretion of catecholamines or catecholamine precursors

- Catecholamine secretion normally occurs with stress.
  - Stress can contribute to disease (e.g., anxiety, hypertension, cardiovascular disease, renal disease), but such catecholamine excess is a consequence of the stress and is not its cause.
    - Therefore, medical evaluation of the patient for catecholamine excess is not appropriate.
- Pathologic elevations in catecholamines occur in the setting of several catecholamine-secreting tumors (e.g., pheochromocytoma and neuroblastoma) when catecholamines should be measured for diagnosis and management purposes.
  - Pheochromocytoma is a catecholamine-secreting tumor of the adrenal medulla (and also may occur extra-adrenally).
    - Symptoms of catecholamine excess bring the patient to clinical recognition (Table 4.6).

Table 4.6 Classical findings in pheochromocytoma.

Episodic hypertension associated with:
Anxiety
Sweating (common in children)
Pallor
Headache (common in children)
Tachycardia
Palpitations
Feeling of impending doom
Nausea (common in children)
Sustained hypertension has been seen in children

- Hypertension from catecholamine-excess in pheochromocytoma can cause:
  - Heart attack;
  - Stroke; or
  - Renal failure

- 10% of pheochromocytomas occur outside the adrenal gland (e.g., in the sympathetic tissue along the organ of Zuckerkandl in a paraganglionic location).
  - 10% occur in children.
  - 10% are bilateral.
  - 10% are malignant.
  - Possibly up to 25% are familial.
- Pheochromocytoma and medullary thyroid carcinoma constitute the type 2 multiple endocrine neoplasia syndrome (MEN type 2).
  - This is an autosomal dominant condition caused by mutations in the RET proto-oncogene.
- Familial pheochromocytoma (or paraganglioma) and some neurocutaneous disorders are genetic causes of pheochromocytoma/paraganglioma.
  - E.g., Neurofibromatosis type 1 (*NF1* gene), von Hippel-Lindau syndrome (*VHL* gene), Sturge-Weber syndrome (*GNAQ* gene), Familial Paraganglioma Syndromes (genes encoding subunits of the succinate dehydrogenase [*SDH*] enzyme complex)
- The best tests for diagnosis of pheochromocytoma are:
  - Plasma free metanephrines or
  - 24-h urine metanephrines.
- Epinephrine and norepinephrine are not as sensitive or specific for pheochromocytoma as metanephrines.
- Can measure dopamine metabolites: HVA (or methoxytyramine which is an intermediate product between dopamine and HVA metabolism) or VMA as a biomarker measured in the urine for neuroblastoma.
- Neuroblastoma, ganglioneuroblastoma, and ganglioneuroma secrete catecholamines, but symptoms of catecholamine excess usually do not occur.
- Neuroblastoma is a pediatric tumor that can even be present at birth (i.e., the tumor developed in utero).

Catecholamine deficiency states

- Catecholamines are essential for survival.
- Excluding people with longstanding diabetes mellitus, catecholamine deficiency is exceedingly rare.
  - This may be explained by the importance of catecholamines in the fight-or-flight response.
- After many years of diabetes mellitus, the normal counter-regulatory release of epinephrine in response to hypoglycemia may be reduced.
  - Similarly, the normal counter-regulatory release of glucagon in response to hypoglycemia may be also reduced.

Conclusion

- The adrenal is a complex gland because the cortex and medulla each secrete unique hormones and the adrenal cortex secretes three varieties of hormones: mineralocorticoids, glucocorticoids, and adrenal androgens.
- Expressions of adrenal disease include hormone excesses, hormone deficiencies, and neoplasms of the adrenal gland.

Suggested reading

Betterle C, Morlin L. Autoimmune Addison's disease. Endocr Dev 2011;20:161–72.

Deipolyi A, Karaosmanoğlu A, Habito C, Brannan S, Wicky S, Hirsch J, Oklu R. The role of bilateral inferior petrosal sinus sampling in the diagnostic evaluation of Cushing syndrome. Diagn Interv Radiol 2012;18:132–8.

Ejaz S, Vassilopoulou-Sellin R, Busaidy NL, Hu MI, Waguespack SG, Jimenez C, et al. Cushing syndrome secondary to ectopic adrenocorticotropic hormone secretion: the University of Texas MD Anderson Cancer Center Experience. Cancer 2011;117:4381–9.

Hassan-Smith Z, Stewart PM. Inherited forms of mineralocorticoid hypertension. Curr Opin Endocrinol Diabetes Obes 2011;18:177–85.

Kamrath C, Maser-Gluth C, Haag C, Schulze E. Diagnosis of glucocorticoid-remediable aldosteronism in hypertensive children. Horm Res Paediatr 2011;76(2):93–8. https://doi.org/10.1159/00032652.

Nimkarn S, Lin-Su K, New MI. Steroid 21 hydroxylase deficiency congenital adrenal hyperplasia. Pediatr Clin North Am 2011;58(1281–1300):xii.

Nisticò D, Bossini B, Benvenuto S, Pellegrin MC, Tornese G. Pediatric adrenal insufficiency: challenges and solutions. Ther Clin Risk Manag 2022;11(18):47–60. https://doi.org/10.2147/TCRM.S294065. PMID: 35046659. PMCID: PMC8761033.

Patti G, Guzzeti C, Di Iorgi N, Maria Allegri AE, Napoli F, Loche S, Maghnie M. Central adrenal insufficiency in children and adolescents. Best Pract Res Clin Endocrinol Metab 2018;32(4):425–44. https://doi.org/10.1016/j.beem.2018.03.012. Epub 2018 Apr 10 PMID: 30086867.

Sperling MA, Angelousi A, Yau M. Autoimmune polyglandular syndromes., 2000, https://www.ncbi.nlm.nih.gov/books/NBK279152/.

Williams RM, Ward CE, Hughes IA. Premature adrenarche. Arch Dis Child 2012;97:250–4.

CHAPTER 5

Puberty and differences of sexual development

Normal physiology

- Puberty is a gradual process where gonadotropin-releasing hormone (GnRH) is secreted from the median eminence of the hypothalamus (Fig. 5.1) that
  - Increases at night,
  - Becomes pulsatile, then
  - Increase during the day.
- GnRH gains access to the anterior pituitary gonadotrophs via the hypothalamic-pituitary portal system.
- Following this, LH and FSH are released in a pulsatile fashion from the anterior pituitary.
- LH and FSH are alpha/beta glycoprotein hormones that share a common alpha subunit, whereas their beta subunits are unique. Thyroid-stimulating hormone (TSH) and human chorionic gonadotropin (hCG) are the two other alpha/beta glycoprotein hormones.
  - In males, LH has its receptor on Leydig cells (which produce testosterone). FSH has its receptor on Sertoli cells (responsible for spermatogenesis) (Fig. 5.2).
  - In females, LH has its receptor on Theca cells (secretes androstenedione which is converted to estradiol by the aromatase enzyme residing in Granulosa cells). FSH has its receptor on Granulosa cells (oocytes) (Fig. 5.2).
- Negative feedback occurs via hypothalamic feedback of sex steroids and inhibin produced by the gonads (Table 5.1).
- Axillary hair and pubic hair in women are the consequence of increased adrenal sex steroid concentrations (e.g., dehydroepiandrosterone [DHEA] and androstenedione) and are not the result of ovarian steroid production. Therefore, puberty in females can be divided into gonadarche (estrogen production and eventual gamete maturation and production) and adrenarche (adrenal androgen production).

Quick Guide to Endocrinology
https://doi.org/10.1016/B978-0-443-14135-5.00006-5

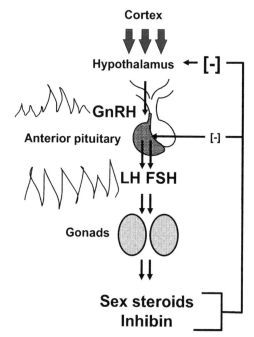

Fig. 5.1 GnRH release from the hypothalamus is regulated by the cerebral cortex. GnRH gains access to the anterior pituitary gonadotrophs via the hypothalamic-pituitary portal system. Subsequently, the gonadotropins LH and FSH are under GnRH control. LH and FSH are responsible for the production of sex steroids by the gonads (testosterone in males and estrogen and progesterone in females) and the production of inhibin. The major site of negative feedback occurs at the hypothalamus. To a lesser degree, negative feedback also occurs at the level of the pituitary. FSH, follicle-stimulating hormone; GnRH, gonadotropin-releasing hormone; LH, luteinizing hormone.

- DHEA is a weak androgen. Its sulfated form, DHEA-sulfate, is present in the circulation in up to an approximate 100-fold excess over DHEA concentrations. Therefore, DHEA-sulfate is technically easier to measure than DHEA.

Males

- Testosterone is the major sex steroid in males.
  ○ It is produced by Leydig cells under the influence of LH (Fig. 5.2).
- Cholesterol is the precursor of:
  ○ Glucocorticoids (i.e., cortisol);
  ○ Mineralocorticoids (i.e., aldosterone);

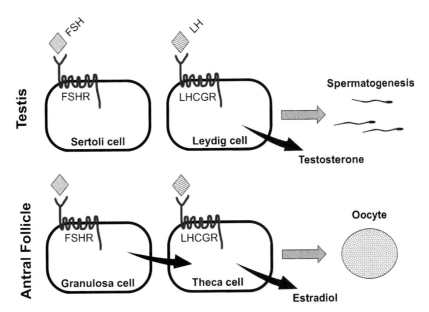

Fig. 5.2 Functionally, in the testis in males and the antral follicle in females, FSH and LH bind to their receptors on Sertoli/Leydig cells and Granulosa/Theca cell, respectively. FSH, follicle-stimulating hormone; LH, luteinizing hormone.

Table 5.1 Hormones involved in sexual development and reproduction.

Hormone	Males	Females
GnRH	X	X
LH	X	X
FSH	X	X
Testosterone	X	
AMH	X	X
Estrogen		X
Progesterone		X
Inhibin	X	X

FSH, follicle-stimulating hormone; GnRH, gonadotropin-releasing hormone; LH, luteinizing hormone; AMH, anti-Müllerian hormone.

- ○ Adrenal sex steroids (i.e., DHEA, androstenedione);
- ○ Testosterone (Fig. 5.3); and
- ○ Estrogen (e.g., estradiol [Fig. 5.3] and estriol)
- The action of FSH is to support Sertoli cells
- Spermatogenesis is dependent on:
  - ○ Tubules (including the Sertoli cells);
  - ○ Spermatogonia;

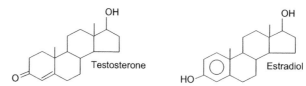

Fig. 5.3 Structures of testosterone and estradiol. Testosterone is produced by the Leydig cells of the testes. In the fetus, testosterone is responsible for the normal virilization of males. At the time of puberty, estrogen, which is produced by ovarian follicles, is responsible for the growth spurt, breast development, and distribution of adipose tissue to the buttocks and thighs in women.

- ○ FSH; and
- ○ Testosterone.
- The testes are outside the abdominal cavity because normal spermatogenesis requires a lower body temperature.
- In males in utero, Sertoli cells produce anti-Müllerian hormone (AMH; also known as Müllerian-inhibiting substance [MIS] or Mullerian-inhibiting hormone [MIH]) that inhibits the formation of Müllerian structures, which are the (Fig. 5.4):
  - ○ Fallopian tubes;
  - ○ Uterus; and
  - ○ Upper vagina.
- Developmentally, local testosterone production by the testes induces the formation of Wolffian structures:
  - ○ Epididymis;
  - ○ Vas deferens; and
  - ○ Seminal vesicles.
- In the external genitalia in fetal males, testosterone is converted to dihydrotestosterone (DHT), which developmentally induces the formation of the penis and scrotum. The enzyme 5-alpha reductase is responsible for this conversion.
- Later, axillary hair and pubic hair develop in response to DHT and adrenal androgens.
- In males, puberty initiation is typically around 11 years old but ranges from 9 to 14 years. Increase in testicular volume ($\geq$4 cc) is considered tanner stage 2.
- Following this, peak height velocity occurs between tanner stage 3–4.

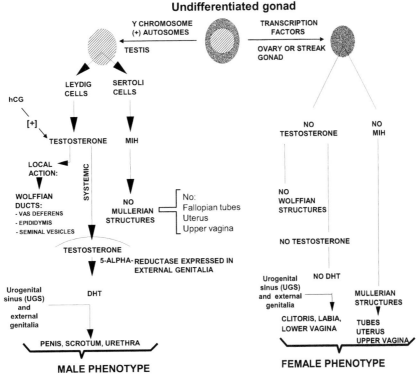

Fig. 5.4 The undifferentiated gonad (center) in utero normally differentiates into a testis or an ovary. Under the influence of Y chromosome genes (including the *SRY* gene) and several autosomal genes, by 9 weeks' gestation, the medulla of the undifferentiated gonad becomes a testis. Under the influence of hCG, the Leydig cells produce testosterone. Locally, testosterone stimulates the development of the Wolffian duct structures (vas deferens, epididymis, and seminal vesicles). As testosterone systemically circulates, testosterone is converted to dihydrotestosterone (DHT) in the urogenital sinus (UGS) and external genitalia to induce development of the male phenotype expressed as a penis, scrotum, and the penile urethra. Sertoli cells within the testicular tubules secrete Müllerian-inhibiting hormone (MIH) that locally suppresses the development of Müllerian structures (fallopian tubes, uterus, and upper vagina). In the absence of the Y chromosome gene expression and the presence of certain transcription factors (the right side of figure), the cortex of the undifferentiated gonad becomes an ovary. If there are not two normal X chromosomes, a streak gonad can develop such as observed in Turner syndrome. In the absence of local testosterone production, the Wolffian duct structures do not develop. In the absence of testosterone and DHT, the UGS and external genitalia develop into the clitoris, labia, and lower vagina. In the absence of MIH, the Müllerian structures (fallopian tubes, uterus, and upper vagina) develop. These events produce the normal female phenotype of the external and internal genitalia. hCG, human chorionic gonadotropin.

Table 5.2 Normal menstrual cycle.

Day	Event
1	Menses begins
1–14	Proliferative (follicular) phase
14	Ovulation
14, 15	Fertilization most likely following intercourse
15–28	Secretory (luteal) phase
20, 21	If fertilization and implantation occur, positive serum/plasma hCG
21, 22	If fertilization and implantation occur, positive urine hCG
28	If no pregnancy, the last day prior to the beginning of menses

hCG, human chorionic gonadotropin.

Females (Table 5.2)

- External and internal genitalia of females develop in utero in the absence of testosterone and AMH (Fig. 5.4).
- The major sex steroids in females during their reproductive years are (Table 5.1):
  - Estrogen (specifically: estradiol) and
  - Progesterone.
- The menstrual cycle is divided into the proliferative (follicular) and secretory (luteal) phases with ovulation occurring in the middle of a normal menstrual cycle.

Proliferative phase of the menstrual cycle

- In menstruating women, estradiol is the dominant sex steroid produced in the follicular (proliferative) phase of the menstrual cycle (Fig. 5.5).
- Theca cells convert cholesterol to androstenedione under the influence of LH. The granulosa cells, in turn, take up androstenedione and, under the influence of FSH, convert androstenedione to estradiol (Fig. 5.6).
- Estradiol causes the endometrium to proliferate.

Ovulation

- Toward the later stages of the follicular phase, a positive feedback loop develops with increasing estradiol levels.
- With the subsequent LH surge (or spike), ovulation occurs with the extrusion of the ovum from the follicle to the outside of the ovary to be picked up by the fimbria of the fallopian tubes. The ovum then travels down the fallopian tube toward the uterus.

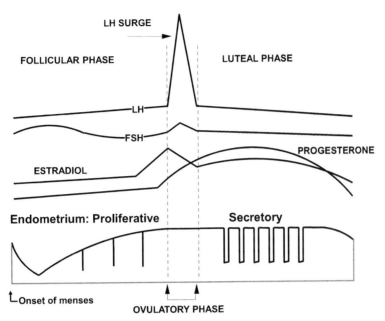

Fig. 5.5 The normal 28-day menstrual cycle begins with the onset of menses on day 1. The menstrual cycle is divided into the follicular phase, where endometrial proliferation takes place as directed by the maturing follicle's production of estradiol, and the luteal phase as directed by the corpus luteum's production of estradiol and progesterone, where the secretory endometrium develops. Toward the later stages of the follicular phase, a positive feedback loop develops with increasing estradiol levels. With the subsequent LH surge (or spike), ovulation occurs (e.g., the ovulatory phase). During the follicular phase, estradiol is the dominant ovarian sex steroid being produced. During the luteal phase, progesterone and estradiol are produced. FSH, follicle-stimulating hormone; LH, luteinizing hormone.

- Some women experience pain at the time of ovulation called "middlesmertz."
  - Essentially, this is the result of a localized area of peritoneal inflammation as the ovum penetrates the peritoneal covering of the ovary.

Secretory phase of the menstrual cycle

- In the luteal (secretory) phase of the menstrual cycle, estrogen and progesterone are both produced.
- Theca lutein cells convert cholesterol to androstenedione under the influence of LH, and the granulosa lutein cells convert androstenedione to estradiol.

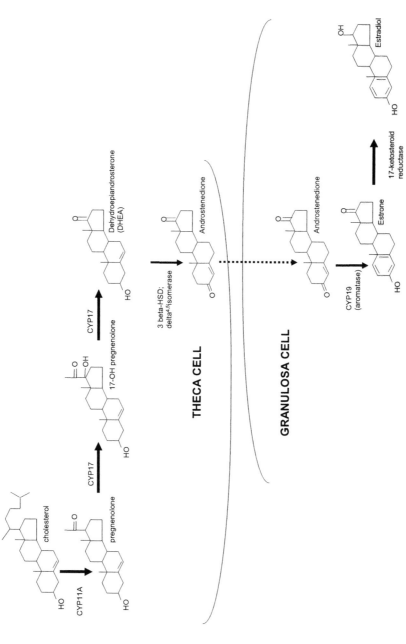

Fig. 5.6 According to the two-cell model of estradiol biosynthesis, androstenedione from the theca cell serves as the precursor for the synthesis of estradiol by the granulosa cell.

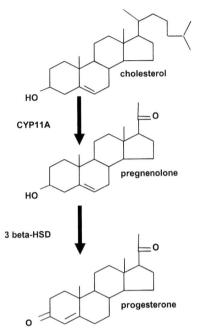

Fig. 5.7 During the secretory phase of the menstrual cycle, the granulosa cell synthesizes progesterone from cholesterol. 3 Beta-HSD, 3 beta-hydroxysteroid dehydrogenase.

- Cholesterol taken up by the granulosa lutein cells serves as a precursor for progesterone production (Fig. 5.7).
  - The granulosa cells respond to LH and FSH.
- Endometrial cells acquire glycogen and there is increased mucus production in preparation for the possibility of implantation of a fertilized ovum.
- Note: Endometrial proliferation does not continue during the secretory phase.

Menses
- In the absence of implantation (and hCG production), the secretory endometrium is no longer hormonally supported because:
  - The corpus luteum becomes the nonfunctional corpus albicans;
  - Apoptosis of the functional endometrium occurs; and
  - Menstrual sloughing is evident and recognized as menses.
- The basalis layer of the endometrium remains and is the source of the functional endometrium during the next menstrual cycle.

Female puberty

In females, puberty initiation is typically around 10 years of age but ranges from 8 to 13 years. Development of breast tissue (i.e., breast buds) is the first sign and termed tanner stage 2.

- Following this, peak height velocity occurs between tanner stage 2–3 with 95% of female growth completed by the time of menarche.

Measurements

- Normal LH and FSH secretion is episodic with pulses every 20 min.
- Ultra-sensitive assays allow for accurate detection of LH and FSH from one sample.
- Prior to ultra-sensitive assays, because of the episodic secretion of LH and FSH, they needed to be sequentially measured three times at 20-min intervals.
  - Alternatively, three samples of equal volume could be drawn sequentially at 20-min intervals and mixed together.

    The frequency of LH and FSH pulses does not change between pre- and postpubertal individuals. However, the height of the pulses changes.
- In women, gonadotropin levels must be interpreted in relation to the woman's menstrual cycle, whether she is in the:
  - Follicular phase;
  - Ovulatory phase; or
  - Luteal phase.
- In children and adolescents, gonadotropin levels must be interpreted in relation to:
  - Age;
  - Sex; and
  - Pubertal stage (e.g., Tanner stage).
- Estradiol circulates bound to sex hormone-binding globulin (SHBG; majority), albumin, or unbound.
- Testosterone is normally bound to SHBG.
  - As testosterone levels rise, SHBG levels decline.
- The free testosterone is the biologically active form of testosterone.
- When total testosterone rises, because SHBG declines, the proportion of free testosterone increases more rapidly than the total testosterone.
- Total testosterone in men is sufficiently high that it can be measured reliably by immunoassay.

- In women and children, accurate measurements of total testosterone require mass spectrometry determinations because testosterone immunoassays usually demonstrate inferior analytic performance in such low ranges.
- In women and children, when androgen excess is a serious clinical consideration:
  - Total testosterone is measured by mass spectroscopy.
  - Free testosterone is calculated with:
    - Total testosterone determination and
    - SHBG determination
- Laboratorians should be aware of the cross-reactivities of sex steroid immunoassays. For example, the estradiol immunoassay may detect Premarin (i.e., conjugated equine estrogens).
- In cases of a differences of sexual development (DSD, see below), steroid measurements should be delayed for at least 48 h after birth because, for many hours after birth, there are high levels of placental steroids in the newborn that can immunologically cross-react with endogenous steroids produced by the newborn.
- hCG is usually quite low (e.g., <5 IU/mL) in nonpregnant women of reproductive age, children, and men.
- Surprisingly, hCG in postmenopausal women can reach levels of 10–15 IU/mL where the hCG is of pituitary origin.
- hCG can exist in a variety of forms that may be of importance in specific clinical situations:
  - Sulfated;
  - Nicked;
  - Free beta subunits; or
  - Hyperglycosylated.
- Plasma or serum hCG assays are commonly able to detect intact (alphabeta) hCG and free hCG beta subunits because various tumors secrete free beta subunits (e.g., choriocarcinoma).
- False-positive hCG immunoassays in plasma or serum have resulted from human anti-mouse antibodies (HAMA).
- AMH can be measured by immunoassay.
- Some clinicians use measurements of AMH as a marker of testicular tissue in newborns when there is a DSD.
- In women of reproductive age, ovarian follicular granulosa cells produce AMH. AMH has been measured as a marker of ovarian reserve.
  - Note: This discussion is beyond the scope of this guide.
- Immunoassays for dimeric inhibin A, inhibin B, and total inhibins are available.

Hypogonadism

- Hypogonadism is deficient gonadal function (Fig. 5.8).
- If the hypothalamic–pituitary–gonadal axis is defective prior to puberty, puberty may be (Table 5.3):
  - Delayed;
  - Diminished; or
  - Absent.

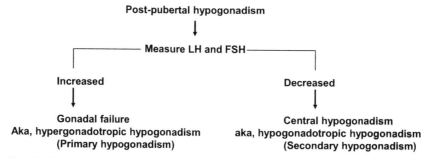

Fig. 5.8 In post-pubertal hypogonadism, there are two general etiologic possibilities. One possibility is that the gonad has failed and does not respond to LH and FSH. Deficient production of sex steroids and inhibin lead to elevations in LH and FSH. In such cases of primary hypogonadism, elevations in LH and FSH (hypergonadotropic hypogonadism) are physiologically appropriate. The other possibility (on the right side of the figure) is that LH and FSH are deficient because of hypothalamic disease (and gonadotropin-releasing hormone deficiency), disease or destruction of the hypothalamic-pituitary-portal system, or pituitary disease. In such cases of secondary (or central) hypogonadism, hypogonadotropic hypogonadism is present because of the deficiencies of LH and FSH. FSH, follicle-stimulating hormone; LH, luteinizing hormone.

Table 5.3 Phenotype of hypogonadism from primary gonadal failure[a] or gonadotropin deficiency[b] in men and women[c].

Onset of hypogonadism	Males	Females
Prepubertal	Absent puberty	Absent puberty
		Primary amenorrhea
Postpubertal	Impotence	Infertility
	Infertility	Secondary amenorrhea
		Premature menopause

[a]Primary gonadal failure: primary hypogonadism, also known as hypergonadotropic hypogonadism.
[b]Gonadotropin deficiency: secondary hypogonadism, also known as hypogonadotropic hypogonadism.
[c]Prior to menopause.

Females

- In females who do not experience puberty, the clinical presentation of hypogonadism is the failure to:
  - Estrogenize (e.g., breast development and adipose distribution to the buttocks and thighs) and
  - Menstruate during adolescence.
    - The failure to initiate menses is termed primary amenorrhea.
- Without puberty, the normal growth spurt in height will not occur.
- Anatomic causes of primary amenorrhea must be investigated by the physician such as imperforate hymen.
- Hypogonadism in females who have experienced puberty is evidenced in:
  - Oligomenorrhea;
  - Amenorrhea; and/or
  - Infertility when pregnancy is desired.
- The cessation of menses prior to menopause in women who have gone through puberty is termed secondary amenorrhea.
  - When secondary amenorrhea is first recognized, pregnancy must be excluded by hCG testing.

Males

- Hypofunctional disorders of the hypothalamic-pituitary-testicular axis in males can present as the failure of pubertal development.
- Without puberty, the normal growth spurt in height will not occur.
- Normally with puberty, due to rising gonadotropin and subsequent testosterone concentrations, there is:
  - Increased testicular size;
  - Increased size of the scrotum;
  - Rugation of the scrotum;
  - Development of pubic and axillary hair;
  - Increased penile size, and the
  - Initiation of spermatogenesis.
- During normal adolescence, erections and ejaculation (e.g., nocturnal emissions) occur.

  Hypogonadism in males who have experienced puberty is evidenced in:
  - Loss of libido;
  - Impotence; and
  - Infertility when pregnancy is desired.

- Adrenarche does occur in males.
  - However, because testosterone is a much more powerful androgen than either DHEA or androstenedione, gonadarche is dominant over adrenarche.
  - Nevertheless, if there is excessive production of adrenal androgens in the prepubertal child (either male or female), pathologic virilization can occur (see below).
- Excessive testosterone (or androgen) administration can cause:
  - Salt retention and hypertension;
  - A decline in high-density lipoprotein (HDL) cholesterol;
  - A rise in low-density lipoprotein (LDL) cholesterol (increasing the risk of atherosclerotic cardiovascular disease);
  - Aggressive behavior (e.g., "roid rage"); and
  - Suppression of LH and FSH, causing infertility and reduced testicular size.
- Certain oral androgens (e.g., danazol, fluoxymesterone, methandienone, methenolone, methyltestosterone, nandrolone, norethandrolone, oxandrolone, oxymetholone, and stanozolol) can produce liver toxicity, including:
  - Liver dysfunction;
  - Liver cancer; and
  - Peliosis hepatis.
  - For these reasons, testosterone itself is administered by intramuscular or subcutaneous injection or topically via gel or patch

Mechanisms of hypogonadism
Primary hypogonadism
- Primary hypogonadism indicates gonadal failure as opposed to hypothalamic or pituitary failure (which represents causes of secondary or tertiary ["central"] hypogonadism).
- With failure to initiate, or loss of, sex steroid and inhibin production, gonadotropin levels are elevated. Therefore, another name for primary hypogonadism is hypergonadotropic hypogonadism.
  - Hypergonadotropic hypogonadism can result from:
    - Developmental disorders of the gonad;
    - Chromosomal defects (e.g., Turner syndrome in females);
    - Defects in steroidogenesis (e.g., 17-hydroxylase deficiency in females or 17 ketosteroid reductase deficiency in males);
    - Defects in the LH or FSH receptor;
    - Gonadal damage from irradiation, chemotherapy, autoimmunity, or surgical removal of gonads; or

- Vascular insults in utero (e.g., disappearing testes syndrome in males).
  - Boys affected with the disappearing testes syndrome are believed to experience infarction of both testes in utero after the time that sexual differentiation to the male phenotype has been completed.
  - These boys are born without palpable testes and do not enter puberty spontaneously because of the lack of testicular function.
- Whether primary hypogonadism presents before or after puberty depends on the etiology of the gonadal failure.
  - For example, girls with Turner syndrome are usually affected with primary amenorrhea because they essentially experience menopause before birth. The absence of two normally functioning X chromosomes leads to disordered oogenesis and there are usually few to no normally functioning oocytes prior to birth.

Central hypogonadism

- Central hypogonadism results from:
  - Hypothalamic failure of GnRH secretion, or
  - Pituitary failure of gonadotropin secretion.
- Disorders of GnRH secretion, the GnRH receptor, and LH and/or FSH secretion indicate a central nervous system (CNS) or hypothalamic/pituitary origin of the hypogonadism.
- Central hypogonadism is also termed hypogonadotropic hypogonadism.
- Any disease affecting the hypothalamus, hypothalamic–pituitary portal system, or pituitary can cause hypogonadotropic hypogonadism. (The spectrum of disorders of such axes was illustrated in Chapter 2.)
- In cases of hypogonadotropic hypogonadism, deficiencies of other anterior pituitary hormones must be sought.
- An appropriate evaluation for hypogonadism in a male includes measurements of:
  - LH;
  - FSH;
  - Testosterone;
  - Prolactin (because hyperprolactinemia can cause infertility); and
  - TSH and free T4 (hypothyroidism can contribute to hypogonadism).

Reproductive disorders in women

- Considering the biologic and hormonal complexity of the menstrual cycle, it is not surprising that disorders involving the secretion of gonadotropins and the response of the ovaries to gonadotropins are very common causes of oligomenorrhea, amenorrhea, and infertility in women.

- In women with oligomenorrhea, if the woman does ovulate, she is potentially fertile. Therefore, if pregnancy is not desired, oligomenorrheic woman should use birth control.
- In women, the hypothalamic-pituitary-ovarian axis can be disrupted by:
  - Psychological stress;
  - Physical stress (e.g., extreme exercise); or
  - Significant weight loss (e.g., anorexia nervosa) or gain (e.g., the metabolic syndrome).
- In polycystic ovary syndrome (PCOS), which is common in women affected with metabolic syndrome, there is disordered gonadotropin secretion and ovarian responses that cause multiple follicles to develop, yet ovulation is impaired or absent.
  - Weight loss and/or use of metformin can often restore fertility. Excessive androgen levels, as seen in PCOS, can contribute to hyperinsulinemia and insulin resistance.
- With continuous estrogen stimulation of the endometrium in the absence of ovulation or progesterone of endogenous or exogenous origin, the endometrium (with or without hyperplasia) can break down and cause irregular menses.
- An appropriate evaluation for hypogonadism in a female includes measurements of:
  - LH;
  - FSH,
  - Estradiol;
  - Prolactin (because hyperprolactinemia can cause menstrual irregularity or amenorrhea); and
  - TSH and free T4 (hypo- or hyperthyroidism can contribute to hypogonadism and irregular menses).
- If hyperandrogenism is clinically present, testosterone and free testosterone can be measured.
  - If the source of hyperandrogenism could be the adrenal gland, DHEA-sulfate, androstenedione, and 17-hydroxyprogesterone (17-OHP) can be measured.
    - 17-OHP is elevated in late-onset 21-hydroxylase deficiency congenital adrenal hyperplasia (see Chapter 4).

Androgen excess

- Postnatal virilization in women is expressed as:
  - Development of male-pattern baldness;
  - Markedly increased midline body hair and beard;

- o Deepening of the voice;
- o Increased muscle mass;
- o Clitoromegaly; and
- o Loss of feminine features (e.g., breast atrophy, a decline in adipose tissue over the buttocks and upper legs).
- Hirsutism (a postnatal diagnosis) is a less severe consequence of excess androgens.
  - o It is manifested as increased midline body hair (e.g., a mustache) without other features of postnatal virilization.
  - o When present in excess concentrations, glucocorticoids can bind to the androgen receptor and cause hirsutism (as observed in Cushing syndrome).
  - o Hyperprolactinemia can also cause hirsutism (via multiple mechanisms including lowering of SHBG and stimulation of testosterone and DHEA secretion).
- If hyperandrogenism is clinically present, testosterone and free testosterone can be measured.
  - o If the source of hyperandrogenism could be the adrenal gland, DHEA-sulfate, androstenedione, and 17-hydroxyprogesterone (17-OHP) can be measured.

Pubertal disorders

Evaluation of pubertal failure

- Nonpathologic-delayed puberty (also known as constitutional delay in growth and maturation) is determined by:
  - o Radiologically measuring the bone age (usually of the wrist) of the child (which will be delayed) and
  - o Seeking a family history of delayed puberty in either parent, although the absence of a family history of delayed maturation does not exclude delayed maturation in the child.
- Delayed maturation is much more common in boys than in girls who present for evaluation.
- In delayed maturation:
  - o The child's biologic clock is slowed compared with typical children, and normal puberty is not expected until the bone age of the child approaches the chronologic age when puberty naturally occurs.
  - o Gonadotropin and sex steroid levels are appropriate for the child's biologic age as indicated by his or her delayed bone age.

- Therefore, hormone levels should be referenced against the bone age of the child and not the child's chronologic age.
  - If the hormone levels are considerably below the reference intervals for the child's delayed bone age, then further work-up may be indicated (see below).
- Physicians may order a GnRH stimulation test to evaluate the hypothalamic-pituitary-gonadal axis when delayed maturation is suspected. However, this is less often performed now that ultra-sensitive gonadotropin assays are available.
  - Failure of any significant increase in LH and FSH following GnRH may indicate:
    - Hypogonadotropic hypogonadism or
    - A normal young child who does not yet express such a response.
  - It is worth noting that the clinician may be challenged diagnostically in these types of cases.
- Although bone age and family history can support the diagnosis of delayed maturation, there are no definitive tests for delayed maturation. Indeed, the diagnosis of delayed maturation is confirmed only when the child spontaneously enters into puberty at a later date than typical age.

Pathologic causes of pubertal failure

- Assuming that the child does not suffer from a chronic disease (that could explain delayed puberty [e.g., severe cases of cystic fibrosis or inflammatory bowel disease]) and there is no obvious cause for the child's failure to enter into puberty (e.g., Turner syndrome in females), gonadotropins and sex steroids are measured.
- If the gonadotropins are elevated, primary gonadal failure may be evaluated (e.g., examined by chromosomal analysis).
  - Other clinical findings may help guide the evaluation.
  - For example, if hypokalemic hypertension is present in a female with who has failed to enter puberty, then 17-hydroxylase deficiency should be considered.
  - Alternatively, this may be a male who is severely undervirilized prenatally because of an in-utero testosterone deficiency or resistance to the action of androgens.
- If the gonadotropins are low, imaging of the CNS and pituitary should be considered.
  - Testing for deficiencies of other anterior pituitary hormones may also be pursued.

- Gonadotropin deficiency is sometimes part of a genetic syndrome involving defects in transcription factors that are critical for pituitary development.
  - In such cases, multiple anterior pituitary hormonal deficiencies can be present.
  - Examples of such transcription factors include:
    - Pituitary-specific positive transcription factor 1 (PIT-1) and
    - Homeobox protein prophet of PIT-1 (PROP1).
- Anterior pituitary deficiencies can result from:
  - Congenital malformations of the CNS (e.g., holoprosencephaly, optic nerve hypoplasia) or
  - They can be associated with facial midline anomalies (e.g., cleft lip, palate).
    Refer Chapter 2 for further information.

Precocious puberty

- There are a variety of pubertal disorders that can be observed in boys or in girls (Table 5.4).
- Precocious puberty (PP) is the development of puberty prior to the normal time that puberty develops.
  - PP is defined in girls as the onset of puberty before age 8.
    - Typically in girls, the first evidence of normal puberty is thelarche (i.e., breast development).
  - PP is defined in boys as pubertal onset before age 9.
    - The first evidence of normal puberty is testicular enlargement, followed by development of pubic and axillary hair and penis enlargement.
- PP can result from:
  - CNS disorders;
  - Pituitary disorders;

Table 5.4 Pubertal disorders in children.

Disorder	Boys	Girls
Delayed or absent puberty	X	X
Precocious puberty	X	X
Premature adrenarche	X	X
Premature thelarche		X
Gynecomastia	X	

- ○ Primary gonadal (e.g., a sex steroid–producing tumor, activating mutation in the LH receptor) disorders; or
- ○ Adrenal (e.g., 21-hydroxylase congenital adrenal hyperplasia [CAH]) disorders.
- In central PP:
  - ○ Gonadotropins LH and FSH are elevated.
  - ○ If there is the question of whether or not the PP is central or gonadal, GnRH testing can be carried out, or basal LH testing with ultra-sensitive assay can be performed.
  - ○ The gonadotropin response to GnRH is pubertal (whereas in PP of gonadal or adrenal origin, the gonadotropin response to GnRH will be limited or flat).
- Central PP can result from any acquired or congenital CNS insult.
- In boys with central PP, concern for CNS lesion (e.g., hypothalamic hamartoma) is high. Whereas, in girls with central PP, idiopathic (unknown cause) is the most common etiology (of exclusion).
- Gonadal (or peripheral) causes of PP include:
  - ○ Autonomous gonadal function (e.g., testotoxicosis in a male).
    - In testotoxicosis there is a gain-of-function mutation in the LH receptor that causes autonomous testicular production of excess testosterone.
  - ○ A sex steroid–producing tumor.
- Adrenocortical tumors can also produce PP through excessive adrenal sex steroid secretion.
  - ○ Alternatively, it is worth noting that adrenocortical tumors may secrete:
    - Aldosterone;
    - Desoxycorticosterone (DOC); or
    - Cortisol (see Chapter 4).
- When a boy postnatally virilizes prematurely, PP is isosexual (e.g., isosexual = same sex, or a boy who virilizes).
- When a female feminizes, the PP is also isosexual.
- By contrast, if a boy feminizes or a girl postnatally virilizes, this is considered heterosexual PP.
- If the adrenal cortex is the possible source of excess androgens, then the adrenal sex steroids (i.e., DHEA-sulfate, androstenedione) should be measured.
- In summary, PP is evaluated by measuring LH, FSH, testosterone (in males), and estradiol (in females).
  - ○ If there is the possibility of an adrenal source of androgen, then DHEA-sulfate and androstenedione should be measured.
  - ○ A discussion of the radiological evaluation of PP is beyond the scope of this guide.

Premature thelarche

- Breast development in a prepubertal girl in the absence of other findings of puberty (e.g., growth spurt, axillary and pubic hair) suggests benign premature thelarche (diagnosis of exclusion) or exogenous estrogen exposure.
  - This could be from foods, creams, supplements or products with phytoestrogens or estrogen-like properties (e.g., lavender or tea tree oil) or medications.
- If the source of estrogen is exogenous, then the breast development should be short lived (or even regress) if exposure is terminated.
- The laboratory evaluation of girls with possible premature thelarche is identical to that of girls with possible PP, i.e., gonadotropins and estrogen should be measured.
- Since males do not normally undergo thelarche, the development of breast tissue in males deserves medical scrutiny.
- Breast development in males is termed gynecomastia, which may be:
  - Bilateral;
  - Unequal; or
  - Unilateral.
- Gynecomastia must be differentiated from increased adipose tissue ("lipomastia") in the breast that may be observed in cases of obesity.
  - In gynecomastia, the glandular tissue and breast bud are palpable and are increased in size.
- A benign, mild form of transient gynecomastia develops in up to 60% of males during puberty but normally regresses following puberty.
  - This is diagnosed by physical examination and requires no laboratory evaluation.
- Assuming that there is no pathologic cause for adolescent gynecomastia and there are cosmetic and social adverse effects, surgery can be considered.
- A variety of drugs can cause pathologic gynecomastia, including:
  - Marijuana;
  - Heroin;
  - Isoniazid;
  - Angiotensin-converting enzyme inhibitors;
  - Tricyclic antidepressants; and
  - Diazepam.
- Pathologic causes include:
  - Inadequate levels of androgens;
  - Anabolic steroid ingestion;

- ○ Estrogen excess or conversion of androgens to estrogens (e.g., Klinefelter syndrome, adrenal tumors, liver disorders);
  - ○ Pituitary tumors; and
  - ○ Malnutrition.
- Estradiol and estrone can be measured in search of excess estrogens.
- Androstenedione can be measured because androstenedione can serve as a precursor for estrone and estradiol.
- Lactation in males is always pathologic. Hyperprolactinemia must be excluded. Males can develop breast cancer. Although breast cancer in males is uncommon (1/100 the rate in women), breast masses in males deserve serious medical investigation.

Premature adrenarche

- Premature adrenarche is the early activation of adrenal androgen secretion in the absence of other findings of puberty.
- In girls, premature adrenarche presents as pubic or axillary hair in the absence of estrogenization.
- The alternative diagnosis in girls with premature axillary and pubic hair is an androgen-secreting tumor of the gonad or the adrenal gland.
  - ○ For this reason, pituitary and adrenal imaging studies are important in addition to measurements of gonadotropins, estradiol, DHEA-sulfate, androstenedione, and 17-OHP in girls who develop premature axillary and pubic hair (see below). Height velocity increases and advanced bone age could also indicate more severe hyperandrogenism.

Girls with signs of hyperandrogenism: Pathologic causes

- If a girl has a classical form of CAH with hyperandrogenism, her external genitalia should be virilized in utero, thus causing a DSD that can be manifested as:
  - ○ labial fusion,
  - ○ rugation of the labia, and
  - ○ clitoral enlargement.
- In cases of extreme prenatal virilization:
  - ▪ The affected female (46,XX) may present at birth as a phenotypic male infant without palpable gonads.
  - ▪ This requires immediate clinical and laboratory evaluation in the newborn period so that the diagnosis of salt-wasting CAH is not missed (which can lead to fatal Addisonian crisis when not diagnosed and treated rapidly).

- Late-onset forms of virilizing CAH (e.g., late-onset 21-hydroxylase deficiency CAH) can produce hirsutism or virilization at the time of puberty.
- In classical CAH due to 21-hydroxylase deficiency, 17-OHP is elevated.
  - However, because the basal 17-OHP is so highly elevated, cosyntropin testing should not be necessary.
  - In contrast, in late-onset 21-hydroxylase deficiency, their diagnosis may require cosyntropin testing.
- Like premature thelarche, premature adrenarche is a diagnosis of exclusion in girls.
  - Androgen-secreting tumors must be excluded as previously discussed.
  - Precocious puberty, premature thelarche, and premature adrenarche in girls are contrasted in Fig. 5.9.

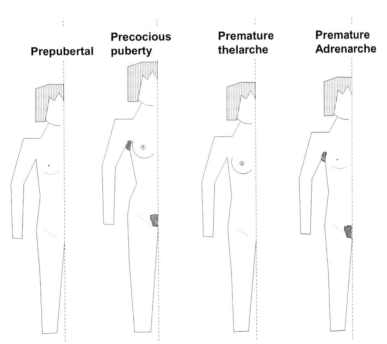

Fig. 5.9 In precocious puberty there is an accelerated linear growth rate leading to increased height compared to peers. Breast development and axillary and pubic hair are evidence of precocious puberty. Precocious thelarche is defined as the development of breast tissue in prepubertal girls without other changes of puberty. Precocious adrenarche is defined as the development of pubic hair and/or axillary hair prior to puberty.

Boys with signs of hyperandrogenism: Pathologic causes

- If premature adrenarche is present in boys, it presents as precocious puberty without testicular enlargement because the adrenal gland is the source of androgen (e.g., the testes are prepubertal in size).
  - Importantly, in such a clinical circumstance, besides an androgen-secreting adrenal tumor, a virilizing form of CAH must also be considered in boys with pubertal changes and small testes if exogenous androgen exposure/ingestion has been excluded.
- As is the case with girls, premature adrenarche in boys is a diagnosis of exclusion.
  - The physician is required to exclude:
    - Inborn errors (e.g., CAH);
    - Androgen-secreting adrenal tumors; or
    - Nonpalpable gonadal tumors; and
    - Cases of PP.
- In a boy with apparent premature adrenarche, an appropriate laboratory evaluation can include measurements of:
  - LH;
  - FSH;
  - Testosterone;
  - DHEA-sulfate;
  - Androstenedione, and
  - 17-OHP.

Differences of sexual development (DSD)

- A DSD is a condition where there can be:
  - Incomplete prenatal virilization of the male genitalia or
  - Prenatal virilization of the female genitalia.
- It can present as ambiguous genitalia where sex cannot be assigned at the time of birth by morphology alone.
- In cases of DSD:
  - There can be a mismatch between the external and internal genitalia or
  - The presence of structures characteristic of the other sex:
    - E.g., a palpable gonad in phenotypic girl or a rudimentary uterus and fallopian tubes in a phenotypic boy.
- The phenotypic expression of a DSD can range from mild to severe, possibly requiring medical, hormonal, surgical, psychological, and psychiatric interventions as well as continuing long-term support.

- Some cases of DSD do not present until adolescence when there may be pubertal failure (e.g., complete androgen insensitivity).
- Because the individual's sex may be difficult to define in cases of a DSD, examination of the patient's karyotype (expedited) guides the current classification scheme.
  - Therefore, DSDs can be classified according to the individual's karyotype (46,XY DSD, 46,XX DSD) or aberrations in sex chromosomes (sex chromosome DSD) (Fig. 5.10).
  - However, the karyotypic information has its limitations because there are 46,XX males (e.g., a sex-reversed male) and 46,XY females (e.g., a sex-reversed female).
- If a gonad is palpable in a newborn with ambiguous genitalia, then that gonad is usually a testis.
- The absence of a palpable gonad does not rule out intra-abdominal testes that have not descended.
- A DSD can result from a genetic mutation or an inborn error of metabolism.
- Alternatively, a DSD can result from a defect in morphogenesis without a recognized genetic or metabolic cause.

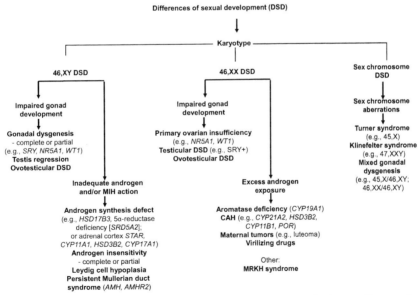

Fig. 5.10 Differences of sexual development (DSDs) are classified according to the individual's karyotype: 46,XY DSD, 46,X DSD, and sex chromosome DSD. See text for details. MRKH, Mayer–Rokitansky–Küster–Hauser syndrome.

- In all cases of DSD, sex assignment will depend on the family's and/or the individual's decision about how the individual will best function sexually, reproductively, and in society based on information provided by healthcare professionals, including:
  - Pediatricians;
  - Geneticists;
  - Endocrinologists;
  - Surgeons;
  - Psychologists; and
  - Psychiatrists.

46,XY DSD

- Individuals with a 46,XY karyotype who have a female, ambiguous, or incompletely virilized male pattern of secondary sex characteristics have not virilized normally in utero.
- In 46,XY DSD:
  - Either the testis fails to form normally (e.g., disorders of testicular development) or
  - There is deficient androgen or AMH action.

Disorders of testicular development

- In a 46,XY individual, the testes:
  - May not have developed (complete gonadal dysgenesis);
  - May have only partially developed, leading to insufficient androgen production to completely virilize the genitalia (partial gonadal dysgenesis); or
  - May have formed completely in utero with complete virilization, yet the testes are absent after birth (presumably because of a vascular accident).
    - Termed "gonad regression" or
    - "Disappearing testes syndrome"
- There may be a DSD in a 46,XY individual with both ovarian and testicular tissue (ovotesticular DSD).
- In any form of ovotesticular DSD, there may be:
  - A separate testes and an ovary on opposite sides of the body; or
  - An ovatestes on one side of the body (e.g., a gonad with both ovarian and testicular tissue) and
  - Either an ovary or a testes on the other side of the body.

Deficient androgen or AMH action

- Androgen deficiency can result from a defect in:
  - The testicular LH receptor (Leydig cell hypoplasia; rare autosomal recessive conditions);
  - The biosynthesis of testosterone (17-hydroxylase deficiency or 17-beta hydroxysteroid dehydrogenase 3 deficiency; Fig. 5.11);
  - The conversion of testosterone to dihydrotestosterone (5-alpha reductase 2 deficiency: the pseudovaginal perineoscrotal hypospadias [PPHS] syndrome); or
  - Resistance to androgen (the androgen insensitivity syndromes).
- 17-Hydroxylase deficiency can cause:
  - Mineralocorticoid excess and hypokalemic hypertension and
  - A female or ambiguous phenotype with intra-abdominal testes.
- The ratios of pregnenolone to 17-hydroxy pregnenolone and progesterone to 17-hydroxy progesterone are elevated (Fig. 5.11).
- 17-beta hydroxysteroid dehydrogenase 3 deficiency is limited to the testes.
- The ratio of androstenedione to testosterone is elevated.
- Various severities of secondary sex characteristic maldevelopment, ranging from an incompletely virilized male to ambiguous to female (female is the most common phenotype), can be observed with 17-beta hydroxysteroid dehydrogenase 3 deficiency.

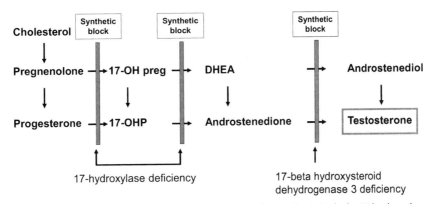

Fig. 5.11 Inborn errors interfering with testosterone biosynthesis include 17-hydroxylase deficiency and 17-beta hydroxysteroid dehydrogenase 3 deficiency. The vertical bars indicate the sites of the metabolic blocks. 17-OH preg, 17-hydroxypregnenolone; 17-OHP, 17-hydroxyprogesterone; DHEA, dehydroepiandrosterone.

- With puberty there are rising testosterone levels and increased expression of male secondary sex characteristics.
- Some affected individuals initially raised as females have adopted a male identity with puberty as virilization progresses.
- Gynecomastia can also develop with puberty.
- In 5-alpha reductase 2 deficiency the ratio of testosterone to dihydrotestosterone is elevated (Fig. 5.12).
- Although such individuals may be initially reared as females, at the time of puberty, with rising androgen levels, the individual can virilize and may change genders from female to male.
- Mutations in the androgen receptor (AR) cause androgen insensitivity.
- Complete androgen insensitivity (CAIS) produces:
  - A female phenotype;
  - Feminization at puberty (e.g., breast development);
  - Primary amenorrhea;
  - A short, blind vagina;
  - Lack of Müllerian and Wolffian structures;
  - Intra–abdominal testes; and
  - Sparse axillary or pubic hair.
- Lesser degrees of androgen insufficiency cause ambiguity or isolated infertility.
- Testosterone levels are high compared to unaffected adult males.

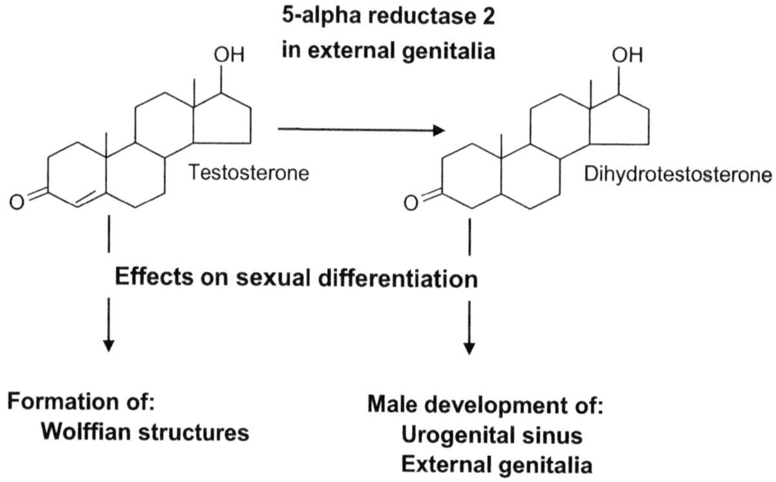

Fig. 5.12 A deficiency of the enzyme 5-alpha reductase 2 (which converts testosterone to dihydrotestosterone) causes the pseudovaginal perineoscrotal hypospadias syndrome.

- Genetic studies of the *AR* gene can be requested from a variety of laboratories.
- AMH deficiency or resistance causes the persistent Müllerian duct syndrome (PMDS; a.k.a.: the "uterine hernia" syndrome).
  - In such cases, deficient AMH action leads to the development of rudimentary Müllerian structures (e.g., uterus and fallopian tubes) in an otherwise normally virilized boy.
- Serum AMH may be detectable in normal girls; however, AMH is at lower levels than in boys up to age 8 years.
- At 9 years or older, there is some overlap in the reference intervals for AMH between males and females (e.g., the high range in females can overlap with the lower range in males).
- PMDS is most commonly discovered when a boy is undergoing surgery for repair of an inguinal hernia and a fallopian tube is unexpectedly discovered. Genetic studies of *AMH* or *AMHR2* genes can aid in diagnosis.
- Clinicians may use the detection of AMH in a newborn as evidence that testicular tissue is present.
- Other causes of 46,XY DSD include:
  - Isolated or complex genitourinary malformations (e.g., exstrophy of the bladder or exstrophy of the cloaca) and
  - Endocrine disrupters.
- Other morphologic anomalies of the GU tract include:
  - Isolated hypospadias;
  - Isolated epispadias;
  - Transposition of the penis and scrotum;
  - Bilateral penis and isolated atresias; and
  - Stenosis or duplications of the penile urethra.
- Endocrine disrupters are environmental pollutants that are believed to cause:
  - Premature sexual development;
  - Delayed sexual development, and/or
  - Disorders of male genital development.

46,XX DSD

- In utero in a female, excess androgens can cause:
  - Clitoromegaly;
  - Formation of a penile urethra (with variable degrees of hypospadias or even a fully penile urethra with the urethral opening at the tip of the phallus);

- ○ Labial fusion; and
- ○ Rugation of the fused labia majora mimicking a scrotum.
- In females, in utero exposure of the CNS to high levels of androgens may result in certain types of behavior more associated with males than females.
- The most common cause of genital ambiguity is fetal androgen excess in 46,XX individuals (Fig. 5.10).
  - ○ This is most frequently due to a 21-hydroxylase deficient CAH (see Chapter 4).
  - ○ In response to elevated ACTH levels because of cortisol deficiency, the adrenal gland anatomically enlarges, thus the term "adrenal hyperplasia" is applied.
  - ○ In individuals with 21-hydroxylase deficiency, 17-OHP is elevated because of impaired conversion of 17-OHP to 11-desoxycortisol, and such precursors of cortisol are then shunted into the synthesis of adrenal androgens, predominantly androstenedione.
  - ○ Cortisol and aldosterone deficiencies due to 21-hydroxylase deficiency can present as Addison disease (i.e., primary adrenal insufficiency) as well as frank Addisonian crisis (see Chapter 4).
  - ○ Less commonly, CAH results from a deficiency of 11-beta hydroxylase.
    - ▪ 11-beta hydroxylase deficiency does not present with salt-wasting (due to the mineralocorticoid effect of elevated levels of DOC) but presents as ambiguous genitalia in girls, with the later development of hypokalemic hypertension.
    - ▪ The 11-beta hydroxylase deficiency in boys can present as hypokalemic hypertension together with precocious puberty.
  - ○ Non-congenital adrenal hyperplasia fetal androgen excess can result from:
    - ▪ Aromatase deficiency (Fig. 5.13):
    - ▪ *POR* gene mutations; or
    - ▪ Maternal hyperandrogenism (e.g., maternal ingestion of androgens or androgenic compounds such as progestins; hyperreactio luteinalis; or maternal androgen-secreting ovarian tumors [pregnancy luteoma] or adrenocortical carcinoma).
      - • Hyperreactio luteinalis results from hCG-driven ovarian theca cell hyperplasia.
    - ▪ Cytochrome P450 oxidoreductase (the product of the *POR* gene) is necessary for normal function of the 21-hydrolase and 17-hydroxylase enzymes.
      - • Defective POR function impairs normal steroid biosynthesis and can cause craniofacial anomalies.

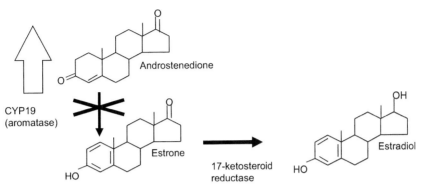

Fig. 5.13 Aromatase deficiency interferes with the conversion of androstenedione to estrone. Estrone is the precursor of estradiol. With aromatase deficiency, androstenedione levels rise, potentially causing virilization of the female fetus.

- 46,XX DSDs can also result from disorders of ovarian development that include:
  - Ovotesticular DSD (46,XX karyotype with testicular and ovarian tissue);
  - Testicular DSD (46,XX karyotype with SRY presence with male genitalia [a.k.a. = a "sex-reversed" male]); and
  - Gonadal dysgenesis or primary ovarian insufficiency (failure of ovarian development with a 46,XX karyotype possibly resulting from abnormalities in gonadal transcription factors *NR5A1*, *WT1*, or others).
- 46,XX males are infertile and are sometimes referred to as "sex-reversed" males.

Sex chromosome DSD

- These types of DSDs involve anomalies of the sex chromosomes, including:
  - Turner syndrome;
  - Klinefelter syndrome; and
  - Mixed gonadal dysgenesis.

Turner syndrome

- 45,X is the classic karyotype causing Turner syndrome.
  - However, this occurs in only ~50% of girls with Turner syndrome.
- Other karyotypes are:
  - 46,X,Xp- (short arm, p arm, deletion of an X);
  - 46,X,rX (ring X carries risk of intellectual deficiency);

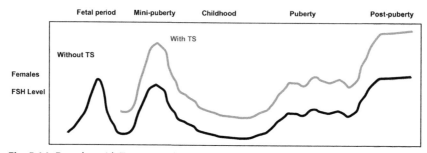

Fig. 5.14 Females with Turner syndrome (gray line) have FSH levels that are higher than girls without Turner syndrome (black line) in mini-puberty, decreasing but not normalizing during childhood, then rising to reach "ovarian failure" levels during puberty. TS, Turner syndrome.

- 46,X,i(Xq) (isochromosome—the q arm is mirrored with absence of the p arm of the X chromosome); and
- other variations.
- Mosaics are:
  - 45,X/46,XX;
  - 45,X/46,X,Xp–;
  - 45,X/46,X,rX; 45,X/46,X,i(Xq); and
  - 45,X/46,XX/47,XXX.
- Girls with Turner syndrome manifest:
  - Short stature; and, generally,
  - Failure to enter puberty because their ovaries involute, becoming streak gonads prior to birth.
  - Other symptomatology is variably expressed.
  - Gonadotropins are high (e.g., elevated FSH) and estradiol is low.
    - Girls with Turner syndrome demonstrate this high FSH elevation both at the time of puberty and during mini-puberty of infancy (Fig. 5.14).

Klinefelter syndrome
- 47,XXY is the classic karyotype in Klinefelter syndrome.
  - These males are infertile;
  - Possible developmental delay;
  - Small testes;
  - Gynecomastia;
  - Elevated gonadotropins; and
  - Reduced testosterone levels.

- Other variant karyotypes causing Klinefelter syndrome include:
  - 48,XXXY;
  - 48, XXXXY; and
  - 46,XX/47,XXY.
- The higher the number of X chromosomes, the more severe the phenotype.

Mixed gonad dysgenesis

- The karyotype is classically 45X/46,XY in mixed gonad dysgenesis, with the individual possibly expressing genital ambiguity.

DSD evaluations

- The complete evaluation of DSDs is beyond the scope of this pocket guide.
  - Nevertheless the laboratory can play a major role in this process.
    - Presently the classification of DSDs focuses on the karyotype, which the laboratory must provide.
- Other key evaluations can include measurements of:
  - Gonadotropins (LH and FSH);
  - Steroid precursors (pregnenolone, 17-hydroxypregnenolone, progesterone, 17-hydroxyprogesterone);
  - Adrenal androgens (DHEA, DHEAS, androstenedione);
  - Sex steroids (testosterone and dihydrotestosterone); and
  - AMH, as well as
  - Genetic analysis of the androgen receptor (if AIS is considered) or *SRD5A2* (if 5-alpha reductase deficiency is considered).
- To maximize testosterone production, testosterone can be measured after hCG stimulation of the gonads (using a variety of protocols).
- Adrenal glucocorticoid and mineralocorticoid evaluations may also be required (refer Chapter 4).

Conclusion

- Reproductive disorders (pubertal disorders and DSDs) are extremely complex and their origins can even precede birth (Fig. 5.15).
- Besides oligomenorrhea, amenorrhea, and infertility in women, and impotence, loss of libido, and infertility in men, there is a wide range of potential disorders affecting newborns (e.g., DSD) or children (early

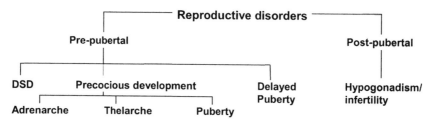

Fig. 5.15 The spectrum of disorders affecting reproduction includes prepubertal and postpubertal problems. Prepubertal problems span differences of sexual development (DSDs), precocious or delayed puberty, premature adrenarche, and premature thelarche. Post-pubertal reproductive problems include hypogonadism and infertility.

or delayed puberty, premature adrenarche, gynecomastia, and premature thelarche in girls) that may involve the adrenal gland or reproductive system.

- CAH is further described in Chapter 4.
- If the source of excess sex steroids is unclear, then cannulation of the draining veins of the gonads and adrenal glands can be undertaken to identify the source and types of steroid hormones produced.
- Developmental, pubertal, and reproductive disorders may originate from systems outside of the hypothalamic-pituitary-gonadal axis, and therefore the astute clinician and laboratorian should keep such possibilities in mind during patient evaluations.
- In the case of an infant with a DSD, sex assignment is an extremely complex and important topic physically and psychologically. Proper sex assignment in cases of DSD should not be rushed; attempting to change the assigned sex of an infant or young child is highly complex and fraught with difficulty.

Suggested reading

Berberoğlu M. Precocious puberty and normal variant puberty: definition, etiology, diagnosis and current management. J Clin Res Pediatr Endocrinol 2009;1:164–74.

Cools M, Nordenström A, Robeva R, et al. Caring for individuals with a difference of sex development (DSD): a Consensus Statement. Nat Rev Endocrinol 2018;14:415–29. https://doi.org/10.1038/s41574-018-0010-8.

Hembree WC, Cohen-Kettenis PT, Gooren L, Hannema SE, Meyer WJ, Hassan Murad M, Rosenthal SM, Safer JD, Tangpricha V, T'Sjoen GG. Endocrine treatment of gender-dysphoric/gender-incongruent persons: an endocrine society clinical practice guideline. J Clin Endocrinol Metab 2017;102(11):3869–903. https://doi.org/10.1210/jc.2017-01658.

Karkanaki A, Vosnakis C, Panidis D. The clinical significance of anti-Müllerian hormone evaluation in gynecological endocrinology. Hormones (Athens) 2011;10:95–103.

Klein DA, Emerick JE, Sylvester JE, Vogt KS. Disorders of puberty: an approach to diagnosis and management. Am Fam Physician 2017;96(9):590–9. PMID: 29094880.

National Institute of Diabetes and Digestive and Kidney Diseases. Androgenic steroids. In: LiverTox: clinical and research information on drug-induced liver injury. Bethesda, MD: National Institute of Diabetes and Digestive and Kidney Diseases; 2012. Available from: https://www.ncbi.nlm.nih.gov/books/NBK548931/. [Updated 2020 May 30].

Rothman MS, Wierman ME. Female hypogonadism: evaluation of the hypothalamic-pituitary-ovarian axis. Pituitary 2008;11:163–9.

Viswanathan V, Eugster EA. Etiology and treatment of hypogonadism in adolescents. Pediatr Clin North Am 2011;58:1181–200.

CHAPTER 6

Disorders related to calcium

Physiology

Calcium

- Calcium is the major constituent of bone and plays an important role in:
  - Neuromuscular and neurologic functions;
  - Intracellular signaling;
  - Cardiac conduction and contraction and
  - Blood coagulation.
- Most calcium in the body is deposited in bone (i.e., ~99%) (Fig. 6.1), while approximately 80% of the body's phosphorus is in bone.
  - The remaining ~1% of total body calcium is distributed between two exchangeable pools:
    - Rapidly exchangeable pool
      - Calcium that has recently been deposited on bone surfaces and calcium that is in the cell cytoplasm, circulation (e.g., plasma), and interstitial fluid
    - Slowly exchangeable pool
      - Calcium in subcellular organelles (e.g., mitochondria, endoplasmic reticulum) and in dystrophic sites (e.g., damaged cartilage, atheromas)

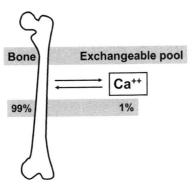

Fig. 6.1 Ninety-nine percent of total body calcium is in bone. The remaining 1% of total body calcium is in exchangeable pools.

Quick Guide to Endocrinology
https://doi.org/10.1016/B978-0-443-14135-5.00008-9

- The plasma ionized (free) calcium that is biologically active is 40–50% of the total calcium in plasma (Fig. 6.2).
  - Otherwise, calcium is bound to anions (~10%) or albumin (~40%).

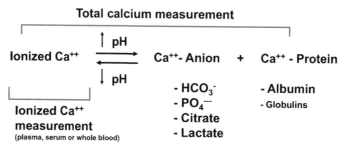

Fig. 6.2 Total calcium is the sum of the ionized calcium plus the bound calcium. Calcium is bound to various anions or proteins. The equilibrium between bound and free (i.e., ionized) is pH dependent. The anions binding calcium are listed, as are proteins that bind calcium.

- The binding of calcium to anions/albumin is pH dependent (Fig. 6.2).
  - In acidotic conditions, ionized (free) calcium rises, whereas ionized calcium declines in alkalotic conditions (e.g., with hyperventilation).
- The ionized calcium concentration is monitored by the calcium-sensing receptor (CaSR), which is a G protein-coupled receptor (GPCR) on the surface of parathyroid gland chief cells (Fig. 6.3).
  - As a transmembrane protein, the CaSR has a large extracellular domain, a transmembrane domain, and an intracellular domain involved in signal transduction.
- Total body calcium is regulated by the absorption of calcium from the gastrointestinal (GI) tract, whereas total body phosphate is predominantly regulated by renal excretion.
- Normally, about 70% of the phosphate absorbed from the gut is excreted in the urine.
- If excess calcium is excreted in the urine (i.e., hypercalciuria), renal tubular injury can follow (e.g., nephrocalcinosis), even causing:
  - Renal failure;
  - Nephrolithiasis; or
  - Both.
  - Urinary excretion of calcium is not a mechanism to regulate total body calcium.

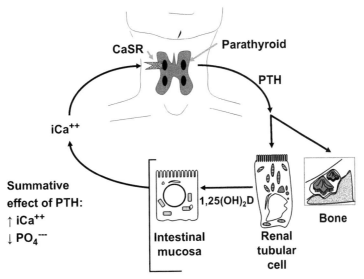

Fig. 6.3 Calcium sensing receptors (CaSRs) on parathyroid cells monitor the ionized calcium concentration in the interstitium that reflects the ionized calcium concentration (iCa^{2+}) in the plasma. Via the action of PTH on renal tubular cells, intestinal mucosa cells (via increased 1,25-OH2D), and bone, calcium levels rise and phosphate levels decline. 1,25-OH2D, 1,25-dihydroxyvitamin D; CaSR, calcium-sensing receptor; PTH, parathyroid hormone.

Parathyroid hormone

- Parathyroid hormone (PTH) is the physiologic hormonal product of the parathyroid glands.
  - Normally, there are four parathyroid glands located behind the thyroid gland (Fig. 6.3).
  - However, there can be fewer than four glands or more than four parathyroid glands located in the neck or chest cavity.
- The CaSR is highly sensitive to fluctuations in ionized calcium and responds quickly.
  - Decreases in ionized calcium concentration elicit the release of PTH from the parathyroid glands (Fig. 6.4).
  - Elevated levels of ionized calcium suppress PTH release.
- PTH is the cleavage product of preproPTH which is cleaved to the intermediate proPTH precursor molecule (Fig. 6.5).
  - ProPTH enters the lumen of the endoplasmic reticulum.

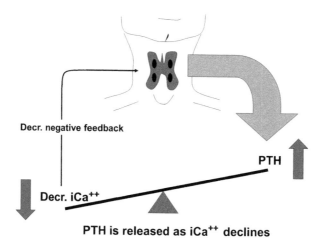

PTH is released as iCa⁺⁺ declines

Fig. 6.4 If iCa^{2+} declines, PTH is released. Via the action of PTH on intestinal mucosa cells (via increased 1,25-OH2D), renal tubular cells, and bone, calcium levels rise and phosphate levels decline (see Fig. 6.2). The increased calcium levels would then feedback negatively on PTH secretion. 1,25-OH2D, 1,25-dihydroxyvitamin D; PTH, parathyroid hormone.

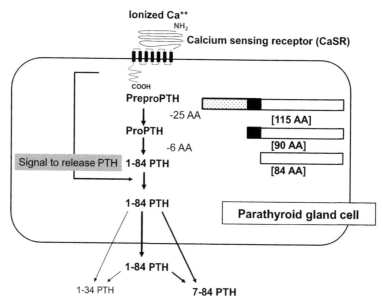

Fig. 6.5 Synthesis of and degradation of PTH. (See text for details.) CaSR, calcium-sensing receptor; PTH, parathyroid hormone.

- ProPTH is then cleaved.
  - Cleavage releases the "intact" 84 amino acid PTH species (1–84 PTH; Fig. 6.5).
- Prior to and after secretion, PTH is cleaved to a 7–84 fragment (7–84 PTH) and a 1–34 fragment (1–34 PTH).
  - The usual ratio of 1–84 PTH and 7–84 PTH in the circulation is ~1:1.
- Presently, PTH is measured by PTH immunoassays (see below).
- PTH has diverse actions (Table 6.1) and while the actions can be summed as increased calcium and decreased phosphorus levels (Fig. 6.3), actions of PTH on individual organs vary (Fig. 6.6).

Table 6.1 Major actions of parathyroid hormone.

Action	Comment
Stimulates bone turnover	Necessary for normal bone health; when in excess causes bone resorption
Stimulates renal tubular reabsorption of calcium	Protective of hypercalciuria, which may otherwise cause nephrocalcinosis or nephrolithiasis
Stimulates renal tubular excretion of phosphate	Overall raises plasma calcium and lowers plasma phosphate via phosphaturia; these actions prevent the occurrence of ectopic calcification
Stimulates increased calcium and phosphate absorption from the gut	Total body calcium is regulated by absorption; total body phosphate is regulated by renal excretion

- For example, the conversion of 25-hydroxyvitamin D (25-OHD) to 1,25-dihydroxyvitamin D (1,25-OH2D) by the enzyme 1-alpha hydroxylase is increased by PTH action at the level of the kidney (Fig. 6.7).
- Vitamin D is a fat-soluble vitamin and requires bile secretion for absorption from the gut.
  - Dietary ergosterol is converted to ergocalciferol (vitamin D2) via exposure to UV light and thermal isomerization (Fig. 6.8).
  - In the skin, 7-dehydrocholesterol is converted to cholecalciferol (vitamin D3) (Fig. 6.9).
  - Dietary vitamin D (vitamin D2) or endogenous vitamin D from sun exposure (vitamin D3) are converted in the liver to 25-OHD (calcidiol) by the hepatic enzyme 25-hydroxylase (Table 6.2) (Fig. 6.10).
  - Measurements of 25-OHD reflect vitamin D stores.

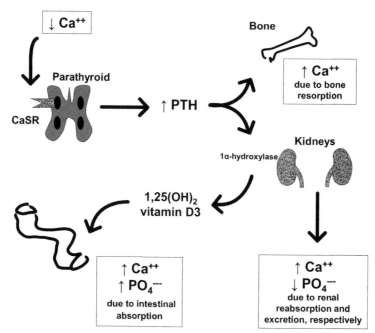

Fig. 6.6 In the setting of low ionized calcium levels, increased PTH release causes increases in calcium from bone, increases in calcium plus decreases in phosphorus from the kidney, and increases in both calcium and phosphorus (via calcitriol) in the gut.

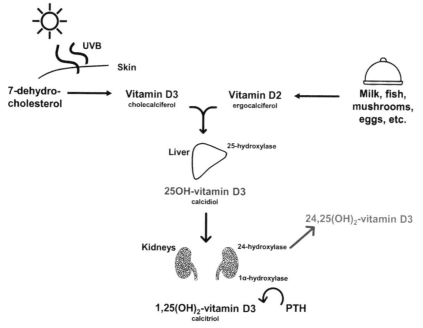

Fig. 6.7 The effects of PTH on renal tubular cells include the stimulation of 1-alpha hydroxylase. This enzyme allows for the activation of the final vitamin D product (1,25(OH)2-vitamin D3). Vitamin D is originally brought into the body via diet or conversion of cholesterol using sunlight. Vitamin D forms in gray are less active or inactive products. 1,25-OH2D, 1,25-dihydroxyvitamin D; 25-OHD, 25-hydroxyvitamin D; PTH, parathyroid hormone.

Provitamin D₂   **Previtamin D₂**   **Vitamin D₂**
Ergosterol   **Ergocalciferol**

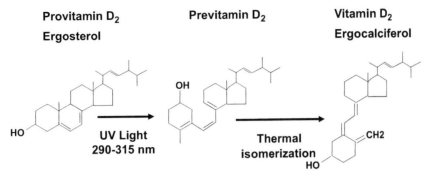

Fig. 6.8 Dietary ergosterol (provitamin D2) undergoes conversion to previtamin D2 when acted upon by UV light. Ergocalciferol (vitamin D2) is then formed via thermal isomerization.

Provitamin D₃   **Previtamin D₃**   **Vitamin D₃**
7-dehydrocholesterol   **Cholecalciferol**

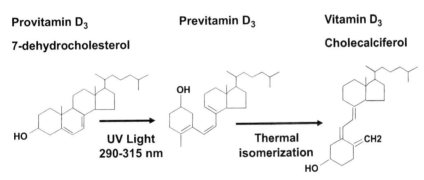

Fig. 6.9 7-Dehydrocholesterol in skin (provitamin D3) undergoes conversion to previtamin D3 when acted upon by UV light. Cholecalciferol (vitamin D3) is then formed via thermal isomerization.

Table 6.2 Vitamin D.

Species of vitamin D	Comment
Vitamin D	Present in diet or develops in the skin from ultraviolet light exposure
25–Hydroxyvitamin D	Produced in the liver from vitamin D; concentrations represent vitamin D stores
1,25-Dihydroxyvitamin D	Produced in the kidney from 25-hydroxyvitamin D; most biology active form of vitamin D

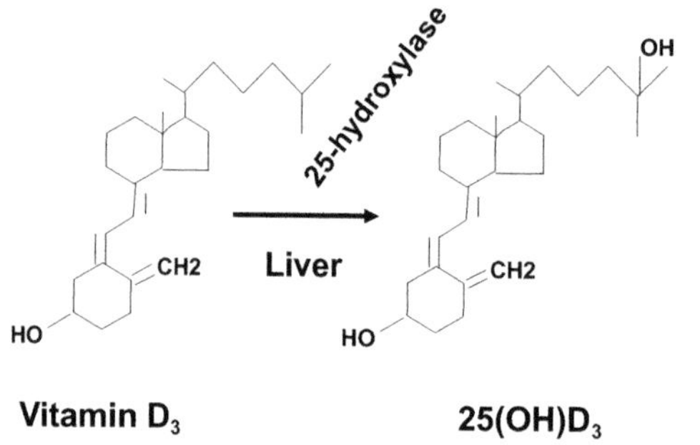

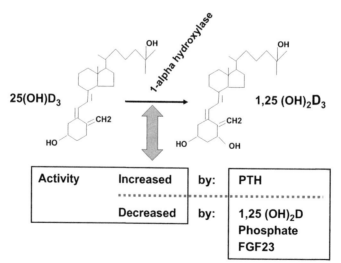

Vitamin D₃   **25(OH)D₃**

Fig. 6.10 Vitamin D is converted to 25-hydroxyvitamin D (25OHD) in the liver by the action of 25-hydroxylase. This process is illustrated for vitamin D3.

- There is no indication to measure vitamin D itself.
- Though 25-OHD is a precursor metabolite it can show some biologic activity.
- High phosphate concentrations, fibroblast growth factor-23 (FGF-23), and high 1,25-OH2D concentrations impair the conversion of 25-OHD to 1,25-OH2D. This conversion is stimulated by PTH (Fig. 6.11).
- Rarely are measurements of 1,25-OH2D necessary.
  - The interpretation of 1,25-OH2D levels can be difficult because a compensatory secondary hyperparathyroidism in states of vitamin D deficiency may raise the 1,25-OH2D level into the low reference interval emphasizing that 1,25-OH2D levels do not reflect vitamin D stores.

Activity	Increased	by:	PTH
	Decreased	by:	1,25 (OH)₂D Phosphate FGF23

Fig. 6.11 Normally renal 1-alpha hydroxylase converts 25-OHD to 1,25-OH2D. The activity of this hydroxylase is regulated by PTH that increases the enzyme's activity in contrast to 1,25OH2D, phosphate, and FGF-23 that impair the enzyme's activity.

- In summary, the renal tubular effects of PTH raise calcium and lower phosphate.
  - The most active form of vitamin D is 1,25-OH2D (calcitriol).
  - Vitamin D stimulates the GI tract absorption of calcium and phosphate from the diet (Fig. 6.6).
- In bone, PTH stimulates osteoblasts.
  - This stimulates increased bone turnover because osteoblasts activate osteoclasts via RANK ligand (RANKL) secretion. RANKL binds to RANK on pre-osteoclast cells causing bone resorption. This process is kept in tight balance by releasing osteoprotegerin (OPG) from pre-osteoblast cells (Fig. 6.12). OPG acts as a dummy receptor for RANKL which prevents RANKL-RANK interaction, reduces osteo-clasts, and decreases bone resorption. This has resulted in valuable drug targets that are discussed below.
  - Osteoclasts degrade (resorb) bone increasing calcium and phosphate concentrations.

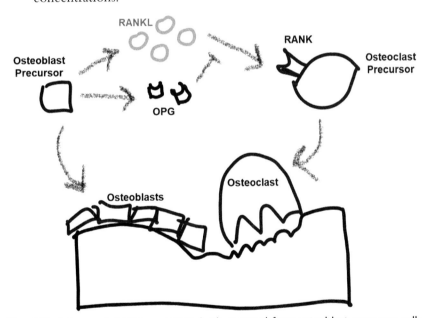

Fig. 6.12 Balance of RANKL and OPG, both secreted from osteoblast precursor cells, maintain balance in bone remodeling as they serve opposing purposes. When RANKL binds to its receptor (RANK) on osteoclast precursor cells, this promotes differentiation to mature osteoclasts. OPG is a "RANK mimic" and can bind up RANKL preventing this process or bone resorption. RANKL is increased by pro-resorptive cytokines (e.g., TNF-α, IL-1, M-CSF production), PTH, and glucocorticoids. OPG is increased by TGF-β and estrogen. RANKL, receptor activator of nuclear factor kappa beta ligand; OPG, osteoprotegerin; TNF-α, tumor necrosis factor-alpha; IL-1, interleukin-1; M-CSF, macrophage-colony stimulating factor; PTH, parathyroid hormone; TGF-β, transforming growth factor-beta.

- Overall, despite increased absorption of phosphate from the diet and increased release of phosphate from bone, the phosphaturic effect of PTH lowers plasma phosphate while plasma calcium rises—as the dominant phosphate response to PTH.
- If the calcium and phosphate concentrations are both high normal and/or high, ectopic calcification may occur. Physiologically, this may be the explanation why PTH lowers phosphate as calcium rises.
- Calcitonin has minor physiologic importance in humans, and a limited role as a calcium-lowering therapeutic.
  - Calcitonin is important in fish to prevent hypercalcemia because seawater (~10 mmol/L) and freshwater (25 mmol/L) contain calcium.
- Phosphaturic hormones besides PTH exist.
  - Fibroblast growth factor-23 (FGF-23) has phosphaturic effects among other mechanisms of action (Fig. 6.13).
    - When present in pathologic excess, FGF-23 can induce rickets or osteomalacia (e.g., X-linked hypophosphatemic rickets or tumor-induced osteomalacia; see below).

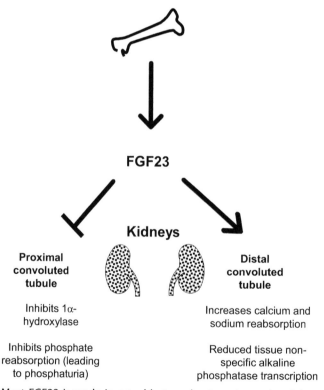

Fig. 6.13 Most FGF23 is made in osteoblasts and osteocytes and mainly acts on the kidney at both the proximal and distal convoluted tubules. The sum effect of excess FGF23 being reduced bone mineralization. FGF23, fibroblast growth factor-23.

Measurements

- Total serum or plasma calcium is measured using a dye-binding assay.
  - Calcium is released from its binding proteins for this measurement.
- Ionized calcium is measured using ion-selective electrodes.
- Intact PTH is most commonly measured by automated double antibody immunoassays (non-competitive assay).
  - These assays actually measure the intact 1–84 amino acid PTH and the 7–84 amino acid PTH fragment (Fig. 6.14).
  - Therefore, measurement of "intact" PTH (iPTH) is a misnomer.
    - There are immunoassays that can selectively measure the "true intact" 1–84 amino acid PTH species exclusive of the 7–84 amino acid PTH fragment.
      - However, in general, such "whole," "true intact," "biointact," or "cyclase-activating" PTH assays provide no significant diagnostic advantage over the routine intact PTH assays.
  - For standardization, calcium, phosphate, and PTH are measured in the fasting state. However, in practical terms, calcium, phosphate, and PTH can be measured any time of the day.
    - Phosphate declines with fasting and will rise with phosphate intake.
  - Hypoalbuminemia can lower total calcium, whereas hyperalbuminemia (e.g., from dehydration) can raise total calcium.
    - Abnormal calcium concentrations require measurement of albumin or ionized calcium.

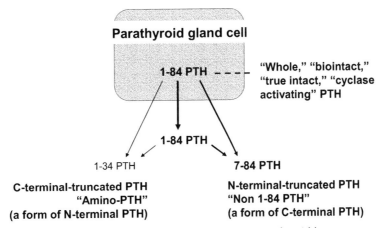

Fig. 6.14 PTH and PTH metabolite nomenclature. PTH, parathyroid hormone.

- In the setting of dehydration with an elevated albumin concentration, hypocalcemia may be masked. In the setting of overhydration with a decreased albumin concentration, hypercalcemia might be masked.
  - As a rule of thumb, the total calcium can be corrected for the albumin concentration as follows:
    - For every decrease in the albumin concentration of 1 g/dL below 4 g/dL, the calcium will decline by 0.8 mg/dL.
    - Conversely, for every increase in the albumin concentration of 1 g/dL above 4 g/dL, the calcium will rise by 0.8 mg/dL.
    - It is not recommended that the laboratory calculate and report such "corrected" calcium concentrations but these are used clinically. It is preferable to measure ionized calcium if the diagnosis of hypocalcemia or hypercalcemia is in question.

Related analytes

- Serum or plasma phosphate should be measured along with calcium when there is a suspected disorder involving calcium.
- Even if the calcium level is normal, phosphate measurements are indicated in several conditions (Table 6.3).

Table 6.3 Indications to measure serum or plasma phosphate.

Renal disease because phosphate is regulated by renal excretion; with a significantly decreased glomerular filtration rate, phosphate rises

Unexplained weakness as hypophosphatemia can produce respiratory failure from diaphragmatic failure

Unexplained cardiomyopathy (cardiomyopathy has resulted from hypophosphatemia)

Malnutrition (for nutritional assessment and the potential development of hypophosphatemia with refeeding)

Use of therapies that can alter phosphate concentrations (e.g., vitamin D, phosphate binders, parathyroid hormone, total parenteral nutrition)

- As noted above, if there is a suspected calcium disorder, either albumin or ionized calcium should be measured.
  - Although it is not as practical, a properly measured ionized calcium level is superior to the calcium level as corrected for the albumin level.
- Disorders of calcium and/or phosphate require a PTH measurement.
  - This is the standard "intact" PTH measurement.

- Biointact PTH measurements (1–84 PTH) are not required for the clinical management of patients with calcium disorders.
- In cases of unexplained hypocalcemia, magnesium should be measured; this is because hypomagnesemia can induce hypoparathyroidism and PTH resistance at the tissues.

Magnesium
- Hypomagnesemia can result from:
  - Inadequate intake;
  - Renal, gastrointestinal, or skin loss;
  - Excessive lactation;
  - Drugs such as cyclosporine A and proton-pump inhibitors (one mechanism can be hypermagnesuria);
  - Acute pancreatitis (theoretically due to magnesium saponification);
  - Massive transfusions or exchange transfusions where citrate binds magnesium; and a
  - Variety of neonatal conditions (e.g., infants of mothers with diabetes, maternal hyper- or hypoparathyroidism).

25-OHD and 1,25-OH2D
- Measurements of 25-OHD reflect vitamin D stores.
  - There is no recommendation to screen the general population for hypovitaminosis D with 25-OHD measurements.
- Measurements of 1,25-OH2D are rarely needed.
  - Some examples of when to consider ordering this activated form of vitamin D measurement include:
    - Hypocalcemia due to vitamin D associated rickets—1,25-OH2D levels can differentiate type 1 vitamin D dependent rickets (i.e., 1-alpha hydroxylase mutation; 1,25-OH2D ↓) from type 2 vitamin D dependent rickets (i.e., VDR mutation; 1,25-OH2D ↑).
    - Hypophosphatemia—1,25-OH2D levels could aid in differentiating genetic FGF23-mediated disorders of hypophosphatemia rickets (1,25-OH2D lower than expected for the degree of hypophosphatemia) from other causes of renal phosphate loss such as Fanconi syndrome (1,25-OH2D normal).

Alkaline phosphatase
- In the absence of pregnancy and intestinal disease, alkaline phosphatase is secreted by the biliary tract and osteoblasts.

- If the PTH is elevated, activation of osteoblasts raises alkaline phosphatase levels.
- Alkaline phosphatase
  - Reflects elevations in PTH and osteoblast differentiation and activation;
  - Is higher in children than in adults by a factor of two- to threefold;
  - Rises after fractures;
  - Is elevated in adults with Paget disease of the bone;
  - Is elevated in the third trimester of pregnancy, where the source is the placenta; and
  - Is normal in osteoporosis (in the absence of fractures).

Urinary calcium

- Measurements can be helpful in distinguishing familial (autosomal dominant) hypocalciuric hypercalcemia from other disorders causing hypercalcemia.
- Although urinary stones are not covered in this pocket guide, urinary calcium is measured in the evaluation of patients with urolithiasis.
- Urinary calcium should be monitored in patients treated with vitamin D or vitamin D analogs (e.g., calcitriol) because hypercalciuria (with its complications) can precede hypercalcemia.
- Urinary calcium can be reported as:
  - A concentration;
  - The absolute amount of calcium excreted per unit time; and
  - The ratio of calcium to creatinine.

Urinary phosphorus

- Measurement of the fractional extraction of phosphorus can be helpful in distinguishing hypophosphatemia as a potential function of familial FGF-23 deficiency or FGF-23 resistance.

Fibroblast growth factor-23

- FGF-23 can be measured when tumor-induced hypophosphatemia is a serious clinical consideration.
- Defects in FGF-23 biology are involved in uncommon types of familial hypophosphatemia with rickets or osteomalacia.

Hypocalcemia

- There are numerous possible causes for hypocalcemia (Table 6.4). Clinical findings compatible with hypocalcemia include:
  - ○ Neuromuscular hyper-excitability (e.g., tetany, positive Chvostek sign, positive Trousseau sign, carpopedal spasm, and muscle cramps);
  - ○ Paresthesia (e.g., "pins and needles" sensation);
  - ○ Seizures; and
  - ○ Prolonged QT interval on ECG.

Table 6.4 Causes of reduced serum or plasma calcium concentrations.

Hypoparathyroidism
Parathyroid hormone resistance (pseudohypoparathyroidism)
Vitamin D deficiency (in its early stages)
Calcium saponification during severe acute pancreatitis (i.e., calcium is bound by the released free fatty acids lowering the calcium concentration)
During recovery from hyperparathyroidism, hyperthyroidism, or hematologic malignancies (i.e., "hungry bone syndrome")
Severe dietary calcium deficiency (rare)
Drug-induced (e.g., bisphosphonates)

- Hypocalcemia affects the sodium channel, reducing the depolarization threshold.
- Basal ganglia calcification and cataract formation can be observed in patients with chronic hypocalcemia.
  - ○ Such calcification may result as a consequence of tissue injury and calcium–fatty acid complexes.
- If the calcium and phosphate are both low, early vitamin D deficiency is likely present.
- If the calcium is low and the phosphate is elevated, hypoparathyroidism or resistance to PTH (pseudohypoparathyroidism) is likely.
- In cases of vitamin D deficiency, the PTH is typically elevated, whereas, in hypoparathyroidism, the PTH is inappropriately low for the degree of hypocalcemia.
- In pseudohypoparathyroidism, the PTH is elevated due to tissue resistance to PTH (Fig. 6.15).

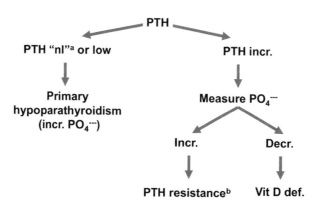

Fig. 6.15 Evaluation of hypocalcemia is outlined beginning with the assessment of PTH. [a]Inappropriately normal. [b]Pseudohypoparathyroidism. PTH, parathyroid hormone; def., deficiency; nl, normal; incr., increased; decr., decreased.

Rickets and osteomalacia

- Vitamin D deficiency produces rickets in children and osteomalacia in adults (Table 6.5).

Table 6.5 Types of rickets (or osteomalacia in adults).

Disorders of vitamin D	Vitamin D–deficient rickets
	Rickets induced by drugs (e.g., phenytoin, phenobarbital)
	Vitamin D–dependent rickets
	Liver disease with vitamin D malabsorption and/or reduced conversion of vitamin D to 25-OHD
Hyperphosphaturia	Familial hypophosphatemic rickets
	Fanconi syndrome
	Other tubular disorders with hyperphosphaturia
	Tumor-induced rickets or osteomalacia (i.e., fibroblast growth factor-23 [FGF-23] secretion)

- In vitamin D deficiency, there is inadequate dietary absorption of calcium and phosphate.
  - The low calcium elicits PTH hypersecretion (e.g., secondary hyperparathyroidism).
  - Elevated PTH raises the calcium back into the lower reference interval, whereas hyperphosphaturia causes hypophosphatemia.
  - The PTH raises calcium through bone resorption, and these elevated PTH levels and low phosphate levels lead to inadequate mineralization of bone and either rickets in children or osteomalacia in adults develops.

- Vitamin D deficiency can result from:
  - Dietary deficiency (vitamin D deficient rickets or osteomalacia);
  - Inadequate exposure to sunlight; or
  - Because vitamin D is a fat-soluble vitamin, from fat malabsorption (called "hepatic rickets").
- Presumably because of increased metabolism, rickets or osteomalacia can be observed in persons taking certain drugs (e.g., phenobarbital, phenytoin) that activate P450 enzymes involved in metabolism.
- Vitamin D–dependent rickets (type 1) or osteomalacia result from an inborn error (i.e., loss-of-function mutation) affecting renal 1-alpha hydroxylase, thus causing a decreased conversion of 25-OHD to 1,25-OH2D.
- Another form of vitamin D–dependent rickets (type 2) or osteomalacia results from end-organ resistance to the effects of 1,25-OH2D.
  - In such cases, there is a loss-of-function mutation in the vitamin D receptor (*VDR*).
  - In this condition, the 1,25-OH2D level is elevated; whereas, in inborn errors involving a decreased conversion of 25-OHD to 1,25-OH2D, the 1,25-OH2D level is low or undetectable.
  - These forms of vitamin D dependency are treated using pharmacologic doses of vitamin D, 1,25-OH2D (calcitriol), or a vitamin D analog such as dihydrotachysterol.
- Rickets or osteomalacia can result from a primary renal tubular defect that causes hyperphosphaturia.
  - Usually a less severe defect in the conversion of 25-OHD to 1,25-OH2D is also present.
  - There are many forms of vitamin D–resistant rickets or osteomalacia in which hyperphosphaturia causes hypophosphatemia.
- The most common form of such vitamin D–resistant rickets (because the rickets cannot be healed using vitamin D alone) is an X-linked recessive disorder that appears to be a defect in the cell-membrane "zinc-metalloendopeptidase phosphate–regulating gene with homologies to endopeptidases on the X chromosome" (PHEX). Such inactivating variants in *PHEX* lead to increased FGF23 expression.
- The treatment of the symptoms of hypophosphatemic rickets has vitamin D and oral phosphate.

    However, in recent years, a monoclonal antibody, burosumab, that blocks FGF-23 can treat the cause of the rickets. Therapy can reduce pain, prevent fractures, and normalize growth.

Inadequate PTH action

- Deficient PTH action can result from:
  - PTH deficiency (hypoparathyroidism) or
  - PTH resistance (pseudohypoparathyroidism).
- These disorders are distinguished as to whether the PTH is inappropriately low (i.e., hypoparathyroidism) or is elevated (pseudohypoparathyroidism).
  - In both cases, in the untreated state, the plasma calcium is low and the plasma phosphate is elevated.
- The causes of hypoparathyroidism are multiple, including:
  - Autoimmunity (isolated hypoparathyroidism or as part of an autoimmune polyglandular syndrome [APS], see Chapter 4 for more information);
  - Genetic (e.g., DiGeorge syndrome);
  - Postsurgical (e.g., following parathyroidectomy for hyperparathyroidism or following thyroidectomy when the parathyroidectomy was unintended);
  - Hypomagnesemia; and
  - Stress-induced hypoparathyroidism (e.g., critically ill patients, including premature newborns).
    - Not permanent and improves as the patient heals
- Pseudohypoparathyroidism can result from defects in the generation of cyclic adenosine monophosphate (cAMP; the second messenger that is normally engaged by PTH) or there is resistance to cAMP (Fig. 6.16).
- The classic clinical phenotype of pseudohypoparathyroidism includes:
  - A round, heart-shaped face;
  - Obesity;
  - Reduced mental acuity;
  - Short fourth and/or fifth metacarpals; and
  - Short stature.
- Isolated individuals and individuals with a family history of pseudohypoparathyroidism who express the clinical phenotype but lack biochemical abnormalities are diagnosed with pseudopseudohypoparathyroidism.
- The treatment of patients with deficient PTH action is activated vitamin D (calcitriol) plus oral calcium.
  - In addition to monitoring calcium and phosphate, urinary calcium should be measured to ensure that hypercalciuria does not develop during vitamin D therapy.

Disorder

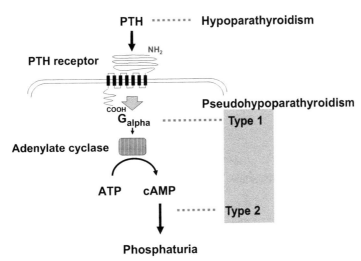

Fig. 6.16 The action of PTH begins when PTH binds to the cell surface receptor for PTH. The receptor interacts with G proteins, liberating Galpha, which activates adenylate cyclase. Adenylate cyclase converts ATP to cyclic AMP (cAMP). A normal major effect of cAMP is phosphaturia. Type 1 pseudohypoparathyroidism involves loss-of-function defects in G proteins, whereas there is apparent resistance to cAMP in type 2 pseudohypoparathyroidism. PTH, parathyroid hormone.

Hypercalcemia

- There are many causes for elevated serum or plasma calcium concentrations (Table 6.6).

Table 6.6 Causes of elevated serum or plasma calcium concentrations.

Hyperparathyroidism (termed "primary" when there is disease of the parathyroid gland itself)
Malignancy
Various non-parathyroid endocrine or metabolic disorders (e.g., Addison disease, hypothyroidism, hyperthyroidism, Paget disease of bone)
Immobilization
Various drugs or therapies (vitamin A or D excess, thiazide diuretics, hyperalimentation)
Milk-alkali syndrome
Granulomatous disease
Recovery from acute renal failure of rhabdomyolysis

- The causes of hypercalcemia can be parsed according to the PTH level (Fig. 6.17):
  - ○ Hyperparathyroidism: PTH is inappropriately normal (within the reference interval) or elevated.
  - ○ Non–hyperparathyroidism causes: PTH is suppressed (which is a normal physiologic response to hypercalcemia) (PTH-independent hypercalcemia).

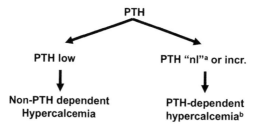

Fig. 6.17 Evaluation of hypercalcemia is outlined beginning with the assessment of PTH. [a]Inappropriately normal. [b]Hyperparathyroidism. PTH, parathyroid hormone.

- Therefore, the measurement of PTH is critically important in the evaluation of any disorder of low or high calcium concentration.
- Because vitamin D deficiency produces a form of secondary hyperparathyroidism, the vitamin D status of the patient should be considered when interpreting the PTH level.
  - ○ If there is any question as to whether or not the patient is vitamin D deficient when a critical PTH level is being interpreted (e.g., in the setting of hypercalcemia), the clinician should consider measuring the 25-OHD level.
    - ▪ If 25-OHD is low, a modestly elevated PTH may reflect vitamin D deficiency.
- Patients with mild hypercalcemia may be asymptomatic. Symptoms of hypercalcemia may be vague and can include:
  - ○ Fatigue;
  - ○ Malaise;
  - ○ Weakness;
  - ○ Depression;
  - ○ Apathy; or
  - ○ An inability to concentrate.

- Hypercalcemia can cause a variety of renal impairments such as:
  - Mild nephrogenic diabetes insipidus;
  - Renal colic from nephrolithiasis; or
  - Renal failure from nephrocalcinosis.
- In cases of hypercalcemia, the following can also be observed:
  - Corneal, conjunctival, and blood vessel ectopic calcification;
  - Bone pain;
  - Cystic bone lesions;
  - Osteopenia; and
  - Pathologic fractures.
- The classic quintet of clinical findings in hyperparathyroidism is:
  - "Bones" (bone pain);
  - "Groans" (GI tract disturbances, i.e., constipation; muscle weakness);
  - "Stones" (nephrolithiasis);
  - "Thrones" (polyuria); and
  - "Psychiatric overtones" (depression, confusion).

Hyperparathyroidism

- The mechanism of hypercalcemia in hyperparathyroidism is predominantly increased breakdown of bone, but there is also increased absorption of calcium from the gut.
- In patients with normal renal function, low normal to low phosphate concentrations result from the phosphaturic effect of PTH, and the PTH stimulation of osteoblasts leads to elevated alkaline phosphatase concentrations.
- Therefore, hyperparathyroidism due to parathyroid adenoma, hyperplasia, or carcinoma (see below) is recognized by hypercalcemia and an inappropriately elevated PTH concentration for the patient's calcium level, low normal to low phosphate levels, and an elevated alkaline phosphatase concentration.
  - In the absence of hyperparathyroidism, when the calcium is elevated, the PTH should be less than 10 pg/mL. However, this is not the case in hyperparathyroidism.
- When there is a primary excess secretion of PTH (adenoma, hyperplasia, or carcinoma), hypercalciuria usually results.
  - When PTH is elevated due to interference in the function of the CaSR, hypocalciuria results (see below).

Brown tumors

- Brown tumors of bone can be observed in cases of hyperparathyroidism.
  - Such tumors are not neoplasms.
- A brown tumor in a person with hyperparathyroidism results from increased bone resorption due to increased osteoclast activity.
  - The width of the bone is expanded (i.e., there is a mass or "tumor" within the bone) and the cortex is thinned.
  - There is increased fibrous tissue in the bone marrow within affected bone.
    - Histologically, the "tumor" is composed of hemosiderin-pigmented macrophages (causing the "brown" color histologically) and multinucleated giant cells.

Primary hyperparathyroidism

- The differential diagnosis of primary hyperparathyroidism can initially be divided into non-neoplastic and neoplastic conditions (Fig. 6.18).

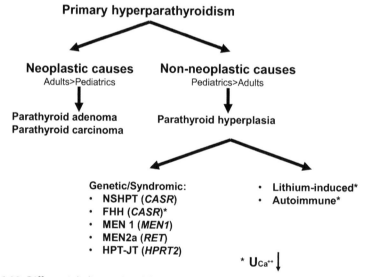

Fig. 6.18 Differential diagnosis of hyperparathyroidism can be divided by etiology (neoplastic versus non-neoplastic) and according to whether the urinary calcium (UCa^{2+}) is decreased. NSHPT, Neonatal severe hyperparathyroidism; FHH, familial hypocalciuric hypercalcemia; HPT-JT, hyperparathyroidism-jaw tumor; MEN, multiple endocrine neoplasia.

o The neoplasms that cause hyperparathyroidism are most commonly benign (i.e., parathyroid adenomas that constitute more than 80% of all cases of hyperparathyroidism in adults and 80%–95% of cases in children) and are far less commonly malignant (i.e., parathyroid carcinoma is present in <5% of cases of hyperparathyroidism in adults). Parathyroid carcinomas are incredibly rare in children.

o The most common non-neoplastic cause of hyperparathyroidism is parathyroid hyperplasia, which usually affects all four parathyroid glands.

- Other causes of non-neoplastic hyperparathyroidism include:
  - Lithium treatment
    o The set-point for negative feedback, as detected by the CaSR, is raised, fostering an elevated calcium concentration due to a rise in PTH. Hyperabsorption of calcium in the renal tubules can also result.
  - Autoimmune hyperparathyroidism
    o An autoantibody directed against the CaSR blocks the perception of calcium by the parathyroid glands, leading to elevated PTH concentrations.
    o The CaSR on the renal tubules is also blocked.
  - Benign familial hypocalciuric hypercalcemia (FHH)

- In lithium-induced hyperparathyroidism, autoimmune hyperparathyroidism, and FHH, hypocalciuria is present because the CaSR on the renal tubules is either relatively resistant to feedback because of a:
  o Genetic error (i.e., FHH);
  o Lithium effect (lithium-induced hyperparathyroidism); or
  o An autoantibody (autoimmune hyperparathyroidism).

- In benign FHH, there is a loss-of-function mutation in the CaSR in the parathyroid gland and renal tubule.
  o This leads to mild hyperparathyroidism and mild, asymptomatic, hypercalcemia.
  o From hyperabsorption of calcium from the urine, there is hypocalciuria.
  o Thus, there are no adverse renal complications from this condition that is, therefore, also known as "familial hypocalciuric hypercalcemia."

- Primary hyperparathyroidism can be associated with:
  o Zollinger-Ellison syndrome (peptide ulcer disease that is the consequence of a gastrin-secreting tumor);
  o Acromegaly; and
  o Types 1 and 2 multiple endocrine neoplasia (MEN).
    - MEN type 1 includes:

- Tumors of the pituitary (e.g., prolactinoma, Cushing disease);
- Pancreatic islets (e.g., gastrinoma, insulinoma); and possibly
- Parathyroids (e.g., hyperplasia).
- MEN type 2 includes:
  - Medullary thyroid carcinoma (where the tumor marker is calcitonin) (100% of cases);
  - Pheochromocytoma (~50% of cases); and possibly
  - Parathyroid hyperplasia or adenoma.
- MEN type 2B is similar to MEN type 2A except that hyperparathyroidism is rare in MEN 2B and patients with MEN 2B have marfanoid habitus (long thin extremities and fingers) and/or mucosal neuromas.
- Primary hyperparathyroidism in a pediatric individual warrants molecular testing due to the higher rate of genetic causes.

Treatment of primary hyperparathyroidism

- Symptomatic patients with hyperparathyroidism require parathyroidectomy.
- Considerations for parathyroidectomy in asymptomatic patients with hyperparathyroidism should take these factors into account:
  - Degree of hypercalcemia
  - There is a previous episode of life-threatening hypercalcemia;
  - Creatinine clearance is reduced;
  - There is markedly increased 24-h urinary calcium excretion; or
  - Bone mineral density is significantly reduced.
- To possibly avoid surgical bilateral neck exploration, preoperative ultrasonography and scintigraphy (e.g., sestamibi radionucleotide scans) are the imaging techniques most commonly employed for localization of the parathyroid pathology.
- If a single parathyroid gland is enlarged, a single gland parathyroidectomy can be performed through a small lateral neck incision, which can be performed as an outpatient procedure.
- For parathyroid hyperplasia, which is more common in children than a solitary adenoma, usually at least three glands are surgically removed and often one-half or one full gland is reimplanted into the forearm to avoid the development of hypoparathyroidism.
- To assist the surgeon in confirming that the biologically hyperactive adenomatous parathyroid gland has been surgically removed, PTH can be measured immediately prior to the neck incision and then again 10 min after parathyroidectomy (because PTH has a half-life of 5 min).

- If the PTH level declines by more than 50% after surgical gland excision, the biologically hyperactive parathyroid has been removed.
- If the PTH does not decline by more than 50%, there may be a second adenomatous gland or hyperplasia may be present rather than a single adenoma.
- If intraoperative PTH measurements are to be made, the patient's neck should not be palpated in the operating room because this can falsely elevate the pre-excision PTH level and may lead to the false conclusion that the correct parathyroid gland was removed when the post-parathyroidectomy decline in PTH was more than 50% *only* because the baseline PTH was falsely elevated by palpation.
- If the PTH has declined appropriately following parathyroidectomy, frozen section study of the excised parathyroid gland should not be required; however, histopathologic examination of the fixed tissues is routine.
- Severe hypercalcemia (calcium >16 mg/dL) is suggestive of parathyroid carcinoma, and anatomic evidence of local tumor spread should be sought (e.g., carcinoma is suggested by a palpable neck mass or parathyroid adherence to adjacent tissues recognized at the time of surgical parathyroidectomy).
- Cinacalcet is an orally administered drug that acts as a calcimimetic (e.g., a drug that mimics the effects of calcium in suppressing PTH levels). Cinacalcet is approved for use in cases of:
  - Hypercalcemia from parathyroid carcinoma;
  - Primary hyperparathyroidism with severe hypercalcemia when surgical parathyroidectomy is not a management option; and
  - Secondary hyperparathyroidism in patients on dialysis because of chronic renal failure.

Secondary and tertiary hyperparathyroidism

- Decreased vitamin D activity due to any etiology can cause a compensatory increase in PTH (e.g., secondary hyperparathyroidism; see the discussion of rickets and osteomalacia).
- Secondary hyperparathyroidism may cause:
  - Bone breakdown;
  - Osteopenia; and
  - Possible pathologic fractures.
- Secondary hyperparathyroidism can cause great morbidity.
  - In addition to decreased vitamin D action as an initiating disorder, a very common cause of secondary hyperparathyroidism is renal failure.
- In renal failure, calcium levels decline because of:

- ○ Hyperphosphatemia (from decreased urinary phosphate excretion) causing calcium–phosphate precipitation and
- ○ Decreased conversion of 25-OHD to 1,25-OH2D (leading to inadequate calcium absorption).
- Secondary hyperparathyroidism of renal failure causes renal osteodystrophy that is manifested histologically as osteitis fibrosa cystica.
- Secondary hyperparathyroidism due to renal failure is treated by reducing phosphate levels through dialysis and/or oral phosphate binders and the administration of 1,25-OH2D.
- As noted earlier, cinacalcet is approved to treat secondary hyperparathyroidism of renal failure.
- Secondary hyperparathyroidism of renal failure should be cured when patients receive a renal transplant.
  - ○ However, if hyperparathyroidism is persistent after renal transplantation, tertiary (autonomous) hyperparathyroidism is present.
    - In such cases, hypercalcemia can develop. Therapy would then be similar to primary hyperparathyroidism, i.e., surgery.

Benign familial hypocalciuric hypercalcemia (FHH)

- FHH is an autosomal dominant disorder involving a loss-of-function mutation in one of the two *CaSR* genes.
  - ○ In essence, there is reduced sensitivity of the parathyroid glands to negative feedback and the PTH rises into the high normal to elevated range, possibly causing mild hypercalcemia.
  - ○ In FHH, the calcium usually does not rise above 12 mg/dL.
- Because the CaSR that is expressed on the renal tubules is also mutated and is relatively insensitive to calcium negative feedback, there is hyper-reabsorption of calcium, thus causing hypocalciuria.
  - ○ FHH in the heterozygous state (i.e., one *CaSR* gene is fully functional while the other gene experiences a loss-of-function mutation) is clinically benign.
  - ○ Lithium-induced hyperparathyroidism and autoimmune hyperparathyroidism are nonfamilial forms of hypocalciuric hypercalcemia.
- Homozygosity for a CaSR loss-of-function mutation is a serious condition that produces potentially severe neonatal hypercalcemia (neonatal severe hyperparathyroidism) that may require aggressive therapy.
  - ○ Craniosynostosis can be a complication of this condition.

Malignancy as a cause of hypercalcemia

- There are two mechanisms whereby malignancy causes hypercalcemia:

- Local osteolytic hypercalcemia
  - The tumor (directly or through local cytokines) destroys bone, which is recognized clinically as the tumor invading the bone. Examples of tumors that cause local osteolytic hypercalcemia include:
    - Metastatic breast cancer;
    - Metastatic colon cancer; and
    - Various hematologic malignancies where neoplastic cells are located in bone marrow.
- Humoral hypercalcemia of malignancy
  - PTH-related peptide (PTHrP) is produced by the tumor and causes the hypercalcemia, but does not cross react in the PTH immunoassay.
  - Immunoassays for PTHrP are available if the clinical question of humoral hypercalcemia of malignancy arises.
- In both mechanisms of malignancy-induced hypercalcemia, PTH is appropriately suppressed because the parathyroid glands are normally functioning. In multiple myeloma, the neoplastic plasma cells activate osteoclasts via their expression of RANKL (receptor activator of nuclear factor kappa-B ligand) including soluble RANKL.

Nonmalignant, non-PTH-dependent causes of hypercalcemia

- Hypercalcemia in Addison disease most likely reflects fluid loss, hemoconcentration, and reduced calcium removal by the kidney.
- In hypothyroidism, reduced metabolism of vitamin D may cause hypercalcemia from increased vitamin D action.
- In hyperthyroidism, hypercalcemia may reflect an increased rate of bone resorption.
- There is increased turnover of bone in Paget disease of bone.
  - Some patients with Paget disease display hypercalcemia.
- Immobilization leads to hypercalcemia.
  - Most likely due to reduced physical stress on the skeleton
  - Similarly in outer space, urinary calcium excretion increases and bone mass declines.
- Pathologic doses of vitamins D and A cause hypercalcemia by increasing bone resorption. Excess vitamin D can also increase dietary calcium absorption.
- Excess calcium in hyperalimentation fluid can cause hypercalcemia.
- Through a high oral intake of calcium and alkali (e.g., in the treatment of peptic ulcer disease), milk-alkali syndrome can result from hyperabsorption of calcium that is manifested in hypercalcemia.
- Although most commonly reported in sarcoidosis, essentially any type of granulomatous disease (e.g., silicosis, berylliosis, histoplasmosis,

tuberculosis) or neonatal subcutaneous fat necrosis can cause hypercalcemia through ectopic expression of 1-alpha hydroxylase with increased conversion of 25-OHD to 1,25-OH2D.

- Acute rhabdomyolysis may initially cause hypocalcemia because calcium is deposited in injured or dead muscle. With muscle healing, the deposited calcium can be pumped out of the tissues, thus causing hypercalcemia.
- Severe and/or symptomatic hypercalcemia in children can be treated with
  - Intravenous isotonic saline as first line to increase urinary calcium excretion (furosemide can be considered as an adjunct if volume overload present);
  - Calcitonin may be used but often only as a short-term remedy due to risk of tachyphylaxis (tolerance develops and the medication becomes ineffective); and
  - Bisphosphonate therapy may be necessary in refractory or severe cases but does carry a risk of hypocalcemia after administration.
- Bisphosphonates act by inhibiting an enzyme responsible for attaching osteoclasts to the bony matrix and thus impair osteoclast's ability to resorb bone (Fig. 6.19). Intravenous bisphosphonates are often utilized in children with bone fragility disorders. A medication used in adults with osteoporosis and undergoing exploration in pediatrics is denosumab, a

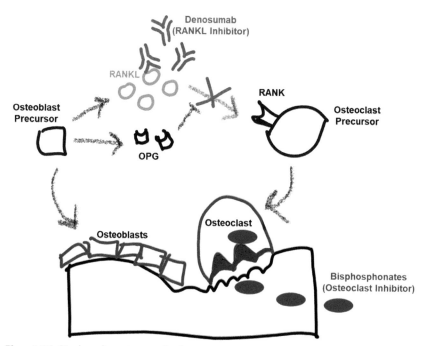

Fig. 6.19 Bisphosphonates and the more recent therapeutic RANKL inhibitor (denosumab) stop bone resorption via targeting of osteoclasts. RANKL, receptor activator of nuclear factor kappa beta ligand; OPG, osteoprotegerin.

RANKL inhibitor, which also inhibits osteoclast function by preventing osteoclast maturation.

Conclusion

- Because of the near ubiquitous effects of calcium on the body, calcium is frequently measured when physicians are faced with patients whose problems are of unclear etiology.
- With a variety of tools (e.g., serum/plasma and urine measurements of calcium, phosphate, magnesium, PTH, 25-OHD), the diagnosis can be narrowed down to direct proper and timely treatment.

Suggested reading

Carneiro-Pla D. Contemporary and practical uses of intra-operative parathyroid hormone monitoring. Endocr Pract 2011;17(Suppl. 1):44–53.

Erben RG. Physiological actions of fibroblast growth factor-23. Front Endocrinol 2018. https://doi.org/10.3389/fendo.2018.00267.

Khosla S. Minireview: the OPG/RANKL/RANK system. Endocrinology 2001;142 (12):5050–5. https://doi.org/10.1210/endo.142.12.8536.

Miller A, Mathew S, Patel S, Fordjour L, Chin VL. Genetic disorders of calcium and phosphorus metabolism. Endocrines 2022;3:150–67. https://doi.org/10.3390/endocrines3010014.

Rodgers SE, Lew JI. The parathyroid hormone assay. Endocr Pract 2011;17(Suppl. 1):2–6.

Unuvar T, Buyukgebiz A. Nutritional rickets and vitamin D deficiency in infants, children and adolescents. Pediatr Endocrinol Rev 2010;7:283–91.

Winter WE, Harris NS. Calcium biology and disorders. In: Clarke WA, editor. Contemporary practice in clinical chemistry. 2nd ed. Washington, DC: AACC Press; 2011. p. 505–26.

Index

Note: Page numbers followed by *f* indicate figures and *t* indicate tables.